475 Herbal and Aromatherapy Recipes

Recipes for life, family and all of your household needs.

Demetria Clark

Note to the Reader: This is an informational guide, a recipe book. It is not meant to prescribe, diagnose or replace medical care and treatment. This book is not inteneded as medical advice, and should not be viewed as such. There are potential risks associated with herbs and essential oils. Because of this, the author, writer, publisher and/or distributors of these book are not responsible for any adverse reactionsor effects associated with any information and recipes in this book. If you have a medical condition or want to use herbal remedies speak to your care provider first. Review all information, research each herb and essential oil before use and do not use something that you feel is not safe or in the proper application.

First Printing: 2013
©Demetria Clark
Heart of Herbs Herbal School Books
ISBN-13: 978-0615871783 (Custom)
ISBN-10: 061587178X
www.heartofherbs.com

DEDICATION

When I think of who to dedicate this first volume of the series, it would have to be all of our Heart of Herbs Herbal School students. Students who are mothers, fathers, doctors, nurses, massage therapists, midwives, professionals, builders, waitresses, truck drivers, and people from all walks of life. Our student body is as diverse as the plants we learn about. To them I am grateful, glad they challenge themselves, myself and each other.

I would also like to acknowledge all of my family and friends who are supportive, optimistic and believe in what I do.
Simply said, I love you.

This book is especially in memory of my grandfather,
Henry Theodore Asselin.
Thank you for all you did, all the love you gave and for believing in me.
I will forever miss you.

Demetria Clark

CONTENTS

Acknowledgments   i

1   Introduction   5

2   Everything Oil   41

3   Everything Bath   69

4   Body Sprays   87

5   Salves, Liniments.... 113

6   Face and Hair   141

7   Tea Blends   141

8   Around the Home   153

9   Resources   164

     Index   175

1 Introduction to Essential Oils and Herbals

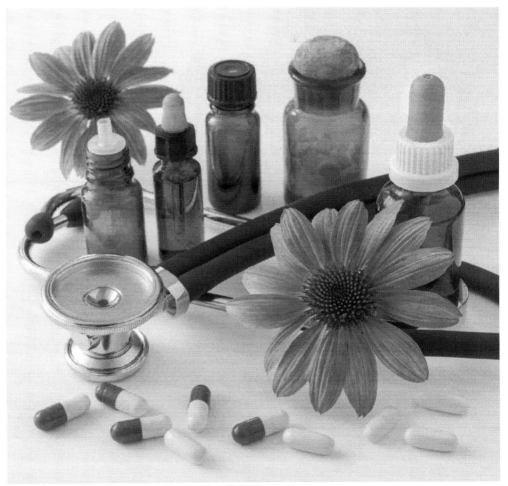

PhotoSGH/Shutterstock

This book is a formulary, not necessarily a how to guide, dosage guide or a herbal and aromatherapy educational manual. We are encouraging the reader to utilize resources if more specific information is needed. If we had provided that for all of the herbs and recipes it would have been a massive book and not an easy to find recipe book. We do have some application and herbal action information, but this is not a materia medica book or educational tome. You will find over 475 recipes and variations listed in this book. All are from my own recipe collection spanning over 20 years. This is not your average herbal, it is not a health book, or glossary of herbal medicine, it is a traditional recipe book.

Most formulations are for external use, household use and overall family use, for use in life. We want herbs to be a part of your life, not just a special part of your life. For hundreds of years homes have had many uses for herbs, not just herbal medicine. All of the uses are very important, and an essential part of the home. Often in modern herbalism we put more weight on medicinal herbalism than household herbalism. I think this is a mistake and further enforces divides and creates a hierarchy in herbalism. I hope these formulas will encourage you to bring herbs and essential oils into your everyday life.

I am a North American herbalist specializing in herbals for pregnancy, birth, postpartum, nursing and children. As a traditional family herbalist, I have worked with families for over 20 years as an herbalist, aromatherapist, midwife, doula and traditional medicine maker. I have worked extensively United States and Europe, blending the two traditions. I lecture and speak at conferences extensively on herbal care for sexuality, pregnancy and woman's health.

I believe strongly in families having options to self-empower and have health and wellness options. I practice what I preach in my books and believe in having a whole family life. In addition I am the author of Herbal Healing for Children, ISBN-10: 1570672148 or ISBN-13: 978-1570672149

More commonly I am known as the Founder and Director of Heart of Herbs Herbal School www.heartofherbs.com and the doula training program, Birth Arts International. www.birtharts.com

HOW TO USE THIS BOOK

Listen to Yourself

Believe and reconnect with your instincts. You know when something is not working for you, listen to your inner voice. If you do not like how something feels, do not use it.

Patch testing skin

A patch test can be done by dabbing, with a cotton swab, a little on a small area on your skin, inner arm, or the back of your knee, and if a reaction occurs then it could be an indication for not using the blend.

Patch Testing the Environment

Before you use something to clean fabric, carpet, tile, porcelain, fiberglass, linoleum, etc.. please test the cleaning formula on a small area. Sometimes discoloration can occur, even though they are generally safe. It is important you test your environment before using. Just because something works for me, or someone else, does not mean it will work for you, or your surfaces. Someone else may have a cotton rug, and yours is wool, many variables exists, so please be aware of this.

Know What is Inside

Know what you are using. Check Latin names, also called Botanical or Scientific names, and look up the herb or essential oil before you use anything. Don't just assume that something will work for you, just because it is listed in a book. Like anything else, remedies, solutions, etc.. are all individual. You are in charge of your own body, so if any of these recommendations cause an interaction or reaction stop using it.

Safety Tips for Essential Oils

1.   Make sure what you are buying is an actual essential oil. Read the label. The ingredients should say for example- Sweet Orange (Citrus sinensis) Essential Oil- Nothing more. Sometimes an essential oil in a store may contain a carrier oil that should also be clearly marked with the oils name. If you are buying a pure essential oil then that is all the product should contain.

2.   Make sure you as the user properly use essential oils. Do not ingest, or apply neat if you want to use safely during pregnancy. This overall is a great rule to follow. I have been using essential oils for over 25 years and I never apply essential oils neat, even "safe ones". This is because I am never sure how an oil will act or react on any person at any time or even myself at any given time. Being careful doesn't mean I don't have faith in the healing attributes, but it means I am aware of the overall power of the plants.

3.   Some oils over time can cause sensitization or allergic reactions. So making sure you never use undiluted oil and alternating the oils you use can assist in preventing that. If an allergic reaction occurs remove the oil the best you can, milk or cooking oil can assist with that. The essential oil bonds to the fat in the milk or oil and then you can shower to assist in further removal. Soaking a washcloth or paper towel in oil or milk and applying to the affected area followed by a bath or shower can assist with removing the oil. I always suggest clients' patch test before using any oil.

   • *Simple patch test instructions, again, said another way, it is that important.*- Apply 1-2 drops of the diluted essential oil to the crease of your elbow, then cover the area or keep it dry for 24 hours. If a reaction occurs then this oil may not be the one for you. Remember that even if an oil does not cause a reaction for you it may for someone else.

   Less is more- In our current world we think more is better, but in reality often that is not the case and it is not the case when working with essential oils. One thing you can always do is use less. If a dosage is 5 drops, see if you get the same results with 2. You do not need to use or make a formula any stronger than you need. Some people get the same results from 1 drop as another does with 5.

Do your homework
Before you buy, and before you use, read about the oil, or make sure it is the one you want. Research the oil, smell it from a few sources, and find the oil you want. Many health food stores, herb shops and essential oil suppliers often have display oils you can smell. Take advantage of these displays and learn about the different scents of these oils. Do not ask a company for free samples. For some reason in the alternative health field we seem to think it is okay to ask for free samples, consultations, lessons, etc... This is not a healthy path to continue on. Most people will not ask a plumber, mechanic, doctor, bookstore, health food store, for free product and services, so please be respectful of the businesses you are working with, just the same way.

Smell the oils
If purchasing oil at a physical location smell the oil samples and make sure you like it. If the oil's scent really turns you off, then find an alternative, listen to yourself. You can always revisit that oil, you did not like at a later date and see if you have the same experience. Often I have at times smelled an oil and thought, "Augh.. Gross" and re-smelled a few months later and loved it, or at least felt differently about the oil. I believe these reactions really have something to do with where we are at a given moment, and listening to what our bodies need. Luckily in almost all cases you can find an alternative oil to support your needs.

Remember that essential oils are flammable. Use caution and care when using them near an open flame, such as a candle diffuser. Read all instructions well on diffusers, vaporizers, candle dispersers, and other type's tools for essential oil dispersal.

Take care to avoid getting essential oils in or on mucus membranes, eyes and genitals. If you get essential oils in your eyes flush them with milk or oil and seek appropriate medical care and advisement. If you get essential oils on your genital areas rinse with oil or milk. You can make a milk sitz bath for vaginal exposure.

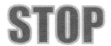

If irritation occurs   using the essential oil blend.

Use appropriate caution when using essential oils with infants, children, pregnancy and elder care.

Never use essential oils internally. Some resources may offer instructions on how to do so, but unless under appropriate care, but since this is a self-care book we are advising no internal use.

Some of these recipes may seem familiar. Some have been included in previous teachings, course materials, lectures and articles online and in my classes. Some of them are from as far back as 1990, some have even been rewritten and placed online. That can occur with recipes, especially with the internet, I have found whole pages of my recipes online word for word, some dating back to original printings in 1998.

Enjoy yourself
Allow yourself to mess up, try again. Herbalism and Aromatherapy are not exact sciences, like all health care options, each person reacts differently and responds differently.

You Are in Charge
As an adult, you are in charge and responsible for your own health. I use herbs exclusively in the treatment of my children, my husband and myself, through illnesses, pregnancy and breastfeeding. I have never been faced with a situation in which herbs have not worked for us, even in acute situations that have required hospital assistance, herbals have assisted greatly in after care and pain management. As an adult your health care choices are up to you, in most situations you can make informed decisions. There can be times when you sense something might not be working effectively for you, or when you feel uneasy about, for example one more round of antibiotics. It is these times more often than not that clients come to me with questions and a desire to try what they consider a more natural and gentler form of treatment. I advise them to be sure to consult their physicians or health care practitioners before changing treatment, and to educate themselves, via books, courses or consulting an herbalist, before

they begin to prescribe remedies to themselves or stop medications or plans their doctors have them on. Most care providers what to do what is best for the patient and they will work with you. Unfortunately in our current medical climate it may not feel that way, but that we have to remember is not the care provider per se but the system they work in, a system we all have to work in to make better.

Essential Oil, Extraction, Storage and Safety

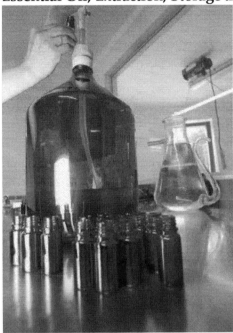

The following is information about essential oils to include hazardous essential oil list. These are particularly dangerous and not appropriate for use, especially by women who are pregnant, nursing or postpartum. These are all the essential oils and not the herbs themselves. A lot of essential oils are not safe for pregnancy are not on this list, this is a list of oils that in general are not safe for use. When an oil is considered not safe for pregnancy, it usually has to do with having an "Emmenagogue" effect, meaning they stimulate menstrual flow, contraction stimulation, they have abortifacient properties (can cause a miscarriage) or can cause harm to the mother or fetus.

Some essential oils have "reputations" for causing one health side effect or another. Many can't be proven with scientific studies or research, but until we have another batch of information we will have to go on the research and information of the day.

Extraction Methods of Essential Oils

These are many different ways to make an extract and essential oil from a plant.

Absolute

An absolute, is not considered a true essential oil, but a classification of its own, but you will often see absolutes being sold side-by-side with essential oils. An absolute is obtained through chemical solvent extraction, and not a true essential oil. Generally the solvent used is alcohol and the alcohol is removed with vacuum extraction. The most common absolutes are Jasmine (Jasminum grandiflorum), Rose and at times Sandalwood (Santalum album).

Enfleurage

This is an ancient manner of extracting essential oils using odorless fats and oils to absorb the critical scent qualities from plants. This method is not as commonly used in modern essential oils. It was most commonly used with plants like Jasmine (Jasminum grandiflorum), Honeysuckle, and other highly scented fatty flowers.

Expression

This method of extracting essential oils from plant material, physically expresses the complete oil from the plant. An example of this is citrus peel when you peel an Orange (Citrus sinensis) you bend the rind, expressing the essential oil from the peel, the liquid the squeezes out is essential oil. This method is also known as cold pressing oils, or cold pressed extractions.

Hydrosol

A hydrosol is the name for the water left after a steam or water distillation of an essential oil. It is mainly water with only a very small amount of water soluble plant constituents. Generally because a hydrosol is mainly water you can use them directly on the skin. Research each one though before using.

Distillation

The most common method of obtaining essential oils is through steam distillation. Remember moonshine stills? This offers a similar idea on how the process occurs. The water is heated to boiling point, and then the steam passes through fresh plant material that has been placed on a rack above the boiling water. The steam and the pressure of the steam is carefully controlled. When the steam passes through the plant material it causes the cell walls of the plants to swell and break down this allows the release of the essential oil. Then the essential oil vapor and water pass through a condenser that cools the steam and the oil into a liquid. The liquid is collected and separation occurs. Most essential oils are lighter than water and collect, or float to the top of the water and they are then siphoned off. Oils that weigh more than water sink to the bottom of the collector and they are then separated.

If you are interested in purchasing your own essential oil distiller you can buy them online, prices vary from about $300.00 to $5000.00 dollars. You can even find instructions online for stills you can make on your own.

Essential Oil Quality
Choosing an essential oil or an essential oil company to purchase from can be daunting. Some basic tips are as follows:

Follow your nose, it may take some time and experience but smelling essential oils is one of the first tips I give for choosing an essential oil. Does the oil smell like the plant part it is distilled from? Can you smell a chemically smell? Can you smell "fillers"? If you can smell chemicals or fillers you may want to pass those oils over.

Read the labels, the ingredients should just be essential oil, unless you are purchasing a blend or diluted blend. We wary of labels that have the words "nature identical oil," "fragrance oil," or "perfume oil." These words may be a sign of that what you see is not a pure, single essential oil. On the label you should be able to see the common name and the Latin plant name, make sure the Latin plant name is the essential oil you desire. Some plants have different varieties as essential oils. For example Orange (Citrus sinensis) oil could be Sweet Orange (Citrus sinensis) (Citrus sinensis) or Bitter Orange (Citrus aurantium). Although that example wouldn't be common it is an example.

Most reputable essential oil companies will offer labeling with more information, instead of less. They want you to know you are purchasing a quality product.

Be leery of terms like "therapeutic grade", "medical grade" or "aromatherapy grade" essential oils. We have no formal standards for these terms and they are being used: Until a standardized description and official grades are made that are universally respected I will tend to not use them to access an oils quality.

Many great brands may have these descriptions or sales and marketing slogans, but overall they are just that descriptions.

As a selling tactic. As a basis for sale, individuals will usually spend more for terms like these whether the quality warrants it or not.

Or as a way to distinguish a product. Although this is not necessarily wrong, as the consumer you need to know that this is not a formal recognition gained to assure quality or purity of the oil. Many in the industry are trying to get rid of these terms because they are confusing to consumers, and some feel misleading.

Fortunately we have no shortage of quality essential oil suppliers and most will answer your questions and welcome feedback from customers. Here are some shopping tips to assist you with your essential oil purchasing.

> *Most essential oils have a year plus shelf life, so that investment is good for at least a year.*

When buying oils make sure it is in a dark bottle, amber is the darkest and I feel really the best, but you can find violet, cobalt and green. They need to have an orifice reducer, not a dropper. Droppers erode from the essential oil and allow air to enter. You need to in addition avoid oils in plastic or clear bottles. Most reputable essential oil companies sell in 4oz. bottles and smaller. Generally a 1 oz. bottle will last you quite a while. Essential oils are not cheap. Look around online and in stores to see what a baseline price is and if the price is too good to be true, then it probably is. In a brief search I found that most organic Peppermint essential oils for an ounce varied from $11-25.00. If you are planning on buying a few oils you can start with smaller sizes and later you can purchase the larger sizes of the oils that you use on a regular basis. So for $100-150.00 you can get a decent assortment of essential oils. I know that this may seem like a lot of money, but to put it in perspective it is not going out to dinner 1-2 times at a nice restaurant in a year or giving up a few activities over the course of a year. You can also buy the oils as needed spreading out the investment. At the end of the book you will find a resource section for essential oils companies that do mail order.

When purchasing online make sure the oils are not all the same price. When you purchase essential oil in bulk to rebottle, they are not all the same price, so selling them for the same price is a little suspect, at least in my opinion. Not all cars can be priced the same, eggs have different prices in the market, and so basic business practices makes this practice of pricing unsustainable.

When at a store looking at a sample, if you put a drop on your finger it should feel clean and not to oily. Essential oils are not true oils like a fruit seed or vegetable oil, so they should not feel greasy. Some of the thickest, darker oils like Vetiver (Vetiveria zizanoides) or Patchouli (Pogostemon cablin) can have a thicker oil feeling than something like Lavender (Lavendula officinalis) or Sweet Orange (Citrus sinensis).

Essential Oil Storage

Essential oils can last from 1 year to many years. Some factors to consider are the type of oil and how they are stored. Here are some simple storage guidelines.

Store all essential oils in a cool dark place. Direct sunlight or light at all will rapidly speed up oxidization and promote breakdown within the oil. I found at an antique store a small cabinet from an apothecary shop that works well.

Often darker colored essential oils have a longer shelf life than lighter colored oils. Lighter colored oils often evaporate faster in air than darker.

Make sure all oils are in dark bottles with a tightly closing cap. Droppers are not acceptable for storage. The bubble rubber will disintegrate in the vapors of the essential oils. If you use a dropper with the oil, you can purchase them separately and wash them between use or purchase extras and have one for each oil. Most oils come with orifice reducers which are small inserts that allow only one drop to leave the bottle at a time.

Shelf life- Most essential oils have a shelf life of two years. Patchouli (Pogostemon cablin) and Sandalwood (Santalum album) can last a few years longer and Tea Tree (Melaleuca alternifolia), fir and Pine (Pinus sylvestris)last about 18 months and citrus oils usually 1 year, longer if they were distilled closer to the time of purchase.

Unsafe Essential Oils
These essential oils are considered unsafe by the overall collective aromatherapy community. Some are because of adverse reactions and others because of overall lack of information. Some essential oils listed do not have any substantial research as to why they are unsafe but they are now part of the collective theory of aromatherapy safety.

Ajowan (Trachyspermum copticum)- Due to the high thymol content it should be avoided in pregnancy. The undiluted oil is a mucous membrane and dermal irritant.

Almond, Bitter (Prunus dulcis var. amara) - Bitter almond oil should never be used in therapy, it contains Hydrocyanic acid.

Arnica (Arnica Montana) - Considered unsafe for pregnancy and most use as an essential oil. Can be safe as an infused oil or homeopathic remedy, and often used as such.

Birch, Sweet (Betula lenta) – The main constituent is methyl salicylate is the active ingredient in aspirin. This should not be in standard use, especially one who is sensitive or allergic to aspirin. It is also not safe for people with liver problems, is on blood thinning medication, or has epilepsy or seizures. It should also be avoided with children or the elderly and while pregnant or breast feeding.

Boldo Leaf (Peumus boldus) - In 2009 the European Medicines Agency assessed boldo as follows: Boldo leaf contains the alkaloid boldine. The 2-4% volatile oil content contains: ascaridole (16-38%), 1, 8-cineole (11-39%) and p-cymene (9-29%). Ascaridole is considered highly toxic, and often referred to as an abortifacient and having teratogenic effects. This essential oil is never considered by any sources in the aromatherapy community that I have seen, to be safe.

Broom, Spanish (Spartium junceum) - Considered toxic from most resources. It is difficult to find decent information, but all resources say to completely avoid the essential oil for all use in aromatherapy.

Calamus (Acorus calamus var. angustatus) - is a newer essential oil and not enough research has been done. It is cited in many resources as not being safe for use in aromatherapy.

Camphor, Brown (Cinnamomum camphora) or Camphor, Yellow (Cinnamomum camphora) - This is not well researched in reference to pregnancy, but in animal studies showed embryotoxic and tetrogenic effects were recorded. Some sources say it has no contraindications, and others state it is toxic and unsafe.

Garlic- (Allium sativa) – Can cause severe skin irritation and in some breathing issues.

Horseradish- (Armoracia rusticana)- the essential oil contains allyl isothiocyanate (as does mustard oil) and is an irritant to the skin, eyes, nose and mucus membranes.

Jaborandi- (Pilocarpus jaborandi) - In some people, pilocarpine can produce vision disturbances, general ill feeling, vomiting, diarrhea, weak heart, respiratory distress.

Melilotus- (Melilotus officinalis) - It is thought that this essential oil contains the chemical courmarin and could be a potential skin sensitizer. Individuals taking blood thinners should also avoid this oil, until more information is known.

Moonwort- (Artemisia vulgaris) - contains a potentially dangerous neurotoxic thujone, it is considered to be toxic, a neurotoxin and potentially an abortifacient.

Mustard- (Brassica nigra) - the essential oil contains allyl isothiocyanate and is an irritant to the skin, eyes, nose and mucus membranes.

Onion- (Allium cepa) - May cause nausea and dizziness, contact irritation.

Pennyroyal- (Mentha pulegium)- This oil should not be used in aromatherapy and even in small doses produces acute liver and lung damage, the oil is a toxin and abortifacient (due to the pulegone content) and if ingested in large doses, the oil can cause death. For years in communities around the country this essential oil has been used to cause miscarriage, the oil was ingested. Ingestion can cause death, liver damage and it is a neurotoxin. We have trained quite a few nurses, EMTs, and other health care officials who first learned about essential oils from the experience of treating someone who had ingested the oil. They wanted to know why, how to prevent ingestion, etc... Please do not ever ingest this oil.

Rue- (Ruta graveolens) - The oil can burn and irritate the skin.

Sassafras- (Sassafras albidum)- This oil can be lethal and it is not safe for use ever.

Tansy – (Tanacetum vulgare) is a toxic essential oils, it is considered dangerous. It can cause convulsions, vomiting, uterine bleeding etc and death is normally the result of respiratory arrest and organ failure.

Thuja- Thuja occidentalis- This oil is not safe in aromatherapy, can cause uterine reflexive reactions and it can cause miscarriage or abortion.

Wintergreen- (Gaultheria procumbens) - can be fatal if ingested. Not safe for use in aromatherapy.

Wormseed- (Chenopodium ambrosioides var. anthelminticum) - This oil should not be used in aromatherapy and the oil may explode when heated or treated with acids.

Wormwood- (Artemisia absinthium) - it contains an extremely high amount of thujone which can be a convulsant and neurotoxin.

These oils can be phototoxic use with care, this means they can cause skin irritation in direct sunlight.

For each of these the effect is really individual.
Angelica Root (Angelica archangelica) stronger effect
Bergamot, expressed (Citrus bergamia) - slight effect
Bitter Orange, expressed (Citrus aruantium var. amara) stronger effect
Cumin (Cuminum cyminum) more of an effect
Dill Seed and Weed (Anethum graveolens)

Stronger Effect- *Make sure you avoid direct sun for at least 3 hours. You may burn.*
More of an Effect- *Avoid the sun for two hours*
Slight Effect- *Make sure you avoid direct sunlight.*
With any of these oils covering up and making sure you don't use them on your face if you are going outside.

more of an effect

Grapefruit, expressed (Citrus paradisi) - slight effect

Lemon, expressed (Citrus limonum) slight effect

Lime, expressed (Citrus aurantifolia) slight effect

Mandarin, expressed (Citrus reticulate) - slight effect

Parsley Leaf (Pertoselinum sativum) - slight effect

Petitgrain Mandarin (Citrus reticulata) - slight effect

Targets oil and absolute (Tagetes minuta, T. glanduifera, T. patula) - Stronger effect.

Tangerine, expressed (Citrus reticulata) - only a slight effect

Carrier Oils

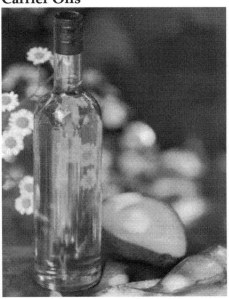

Carrier oils are also referred to as base oils or vegetable oils are used to dilute essential oils, CO_2s and absolutes before applying to the skin. They "carry" the essential oil onto the skin. Different carrier oils offer different properties and the choice of carrier oil can depend on the therapeutic benefit being sought.

Carrier oils are generally cold-pressed vegetable oils derived from the fatty portions of the plant. Unlike essential oils that evaporate and have a concentrated aroma, carrier oils do not evaporate or impart their aroma as strongly as essential oils.

Examples of carrier oils are sweet almond, apricot kernel, grape seed, avocado, peanut, olive, pecan, macadamia nut, sesame, evening primrose, walnut and wheat germ. Most oils bought in the grocery store are not cold-pressed, but instead are heated thus losing their therapeutic benefit. Mineral oil is not used in aromatherapy since mineral oil is not a natural product. It is also said that mineral oil can prevent essential oil absorption into the skin. Mineral oil has also been said to worsen skin conditions and prevent moisture absorption.

Unlike essential oils that do not go rancid, carrier oils can go rancid. Carrier oils that you purchase should be natural and unadulterated. Exceptions include buying carrier oils that have natural vitamin E added because vitamin E acts as a natural preservative. Try "playing" with different types of carrier oils. This will allow you to learn the oil's profile, feel and what it can best be used for.

Please stay away from genetically modified oils and keep the planet in mind when purchasing these items.

HERBS

BUYING HERBS- Always buy organically grown herbs. Try to buy local herbs whenever possible. Herb growers are everywhere, you just have to look around.

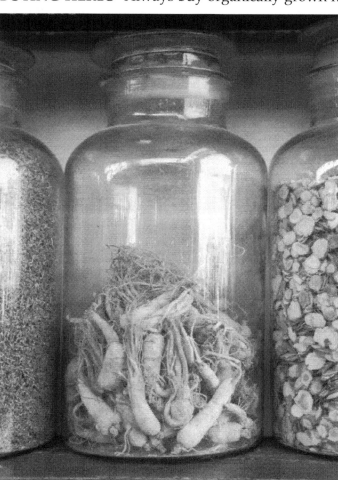

Most large herb companies fumigate their plants because pests could wipe out their entire stock. Many companies also have begun to irradiate their herbs to kill pests, especially if they are coming from overseas. Herbs face importation issues just like produce does. Buying herbs from a distributor who uses overseas suppliers increases your chances of getting . irradiated and fumigated products. While I understand the need to protect stock and follow laws governing import, I do because of these regulations purchase herbs as locally as possible. Many companies are trying to implore safer and more natural means of stock protection.

Using chemically free herbs is as important as eating chemically free foods, but not just for our personal health. When we choose organics, we promote sustainable farming and biodiversity, help reduce pollution, protect the soil and water, and make work safer for farmers and farm workers. Think how much better you will feel, not just physically but emotionally, when you nourish your body and your family with clean, honorably produced food. When we make choices that protect our environment, we are also making choices that protect our bodies.

Buying locally supports your neighbors and smaller farms. Shop for organic herbs at your farmer's market, this is also a great place to get starter plants for your garden, vegetables, fruits and herbs. Get to know the people who grow them. When I buy garlic or Echinacea plants from the farmer down the road, I know I'm getting fresh and potent garlic, and strong local Echinacea, and that will do its job in my remedies.

Buying locally fosters community, directly makes a difference in your local economy and lessens your carbon footprint.

If you can't buy locally, seek out organic herbs and herbal products at natural-food stores—usually in the bulk section—or from specialty retailers. Research your sources.

GROWING YOUR OWN HERBS

Gardening books may feature elaborate herbal knot gardens that look complicated and intimidating, but the fact is, herbs are easy to grow. And they can be grown just about anywhere there is good soil, sunshine, and water (and maybe a little compost once in a while). You can grow herbs in a small plot in the yard; in a corner of your garden; or in pots on your porch, patio, or kitchen window sill.

Basic information about growing herbs can be found in almost any gardening book. You can also ask local gardeners, and herb vendors at the farmers' market. These resources can really help you in learning what grows well in your area.

Many will have excellent tips that work in your area, how to work your soil and what varieties do really well in your area. When we moved to NC it was the first time I had a garden with lots of clay, having neighbors who gardened and a good relationship with the farmers at the market really was helpful in getting tips for my region. I had gardens in Vermont, New York and Switzerland, but all climates and soils are different, so having insider information is so beneficial.

When planting your herb garden, try to plant from seeds as much as possible. This saves money, of course, and it also teaches you about gardening and what grows well in your area. Don't be concerned with straight-as-an-arrow row planting or pulling every last weed. Gardening is supposed to be a fun stress reliever. Just trust in the process and allow yourself to observe the journey from seed to harvest.

Wildcrafting simply means gathering plants from the wild—from fields, meadows, mountainsides, natural areas, pastures, or anywhere you can legally pick herbs. If you are not on public lands, request permission from the property owner. This a good way to give herbalist a bad name in a community. Many people skip this step, and don't ask, that is a great way to get someone mad at you. Most people in my experience are tickled to let you pick wild plants from their pastures, fields and woods, as long as you are polite, respectful to them and the land. You never know you may also make a new friend.

Never harvest more than you can use, and never deplete a local plant stand. I often tell my students not to pick more than 10 percent of an existing herbal stand or patch. (However, that percentage can vary depending on the size of the patch.) Other people in the community may also want to harvest the plants. Also consider that animals and insects rely on plants for food, pollination, and other necessities.

Do not pick protected plants. Find out which plants are protected in your area and use a good field guide to identify them. Just because a plant appears to be plentiful does not automatically mean you can pick it. And a plant that is not protected in one area may be protected in another, so find out which plants are protected wherever you wildcraft. If in doubt, don't harvest the plant. Information about protected plants can be found on state wildlife websites (most will have a link to this information) and the USDA website at http://plants.usda.gov/threat.html.

Ways to Use Herbs
Tea

Tea is the use of water and herbs to make an extraction. Water in the case of tea is the solvent. Teas are used for refreshment and as beverages. You can also make a medicinal tea. Medicinal teas are made the same way as infusions and decoctions.

Infusion

Infusions use the more fragile parts of plants, like leaves and flowers. There are few exceptions to this and Valerian (Valeriana officinalis) is one root prepared as an infusion because of its high volatile oil content. This involves pouring boiling water over the plant matter and allowing the matter to infuse. A medicinal infusion steeps for 20 minutes - overnight.

I really like to let my infusions steep for a generous amount of time. I like to allow steeping to occur for about an hour, others only steep for 20 minutes, and it is a personal choice. If it is an herbal tea I really want to enjoy hot I add it to a thermos, or insulated cup to keep it warm.

It is really important to me that they are medicinally potent because I suggest teas for so many tonic and medicinal uses.

Brewing Guide

Type of Tea	Temperature	Steeping Time
Black Tea	212 F or Boiling	3-5 Minutes Steeping Time
Green or White Tea	170-185 F	3-5 Minutes Steeping Time
Oolong	185-210 F	4-7 Minutes Steeping Time
Herbal Teas	212 F or Boiling	5-10 Minutes
Herbal Infusions		At least 20 minutes. Preferably at least an hour.

These are just guidelines, but it is important to be patient and allow tea to properly steep. If it becomes cool and you want it warm, just rewarm before drinking.

Decoctions- This is the method used to get the plant healing constituents from more tenacious plant material such as bark, root or nuts. This is simmered gently with the herb in the water for 20 minutes.

For pre-blended roots and leaves the decoction is the preferred method of preparation. The same goes for a decoction: I really like to let my infusions steep for a generous amount of time.

It is really important to me that they are medicinally potent because I suggest teas for so many tonic and medicinal uses.

Amounts of herb used for decoction or infusion: 1 tablespoon dried herb per cup of water, or two tablespoons fresh herb per cup of water. Teas can be made by the quart and refrigerated for daily consumption.

I often make large jars of tea to have around all day to drink from or to pour from. Infusions and decoctions when made in bulk need to be stored in the refrigerator, and then only for 48 hours at the most.

Nervous System Tea-simple tea recipe
1 part Valerian (Valeriana officinalis) root
1 part Skullcap (Scutellaria lateriflora) herb
1 part Hops (Humulus lupulus) flower
1 part Spearmint (Mentha spicata) leaf
Honey to taste
Prepare as an infusion
You can drink 3-6 cups a day.

Liniments
A liniment is an herbal extraction that is rubbed into the skin. Liniments are used for sore muscles, strains, arthritis, and inflammations or the muscles, ligaments and tendons. A liniment is usually herb and a solvent such as alcohol, vinegar or oil.

To make a liniment for sore muscles for example one would place 4 oz. Of Peppermint in a jar that is 16 oz. Also add 4 oz. Of Eucalyptus. Add a pint of alcohol, or vinegar. Do not use rubbing alcohol, use Vodka. Place in a nice dry place for 14 days and shake twice a day. Then use on the affected areas. You can also add a few drops of essential oil like Rosemary, Peppermint or Eucalyptus.

For an instant liniment for muscle pain is this

½ cup alcohol, vodka will work.

1-teaspoon Peppermint (Mentha piperita) essential oil, eucalyptus or Rosemary (Rosmarinus officinalis) oil. You should first try using less essential oil at first and find the amount that works for you.

Extracts

Extracts can be very easy to make, and a very convenient way to take herbs. First off place as much herb as you want into a glass jar. Then add your alcohol. I usually add three fingers higher than the herb (dried herb) and two fingers higher than fresh herb. Close the jar and allow it to sit in the sunlight for a few days to soak in the solar healing power of the sun and then put it away until done. If it is macerating during a full moon put it outside to gather the moon's energy also. I also allow my extracts to sit for over four months. Many people only allow them to sit for a few weeks to a month. This is not something I advise. I believe an extract should be made to offer the most healing benefits.

Some herbs as we will learn are best made into teas rather than extracts. An easy formula to follow for making herbal medicine is the simplers' method, this method is based on ratios, and the measurements are referred to as "parts". For example 3 parts Alfalfa (Medicago sativa), 1 part nettle, 2 parts raspberry, is a very common 3:1:2 synergy. This simple way of measurement lets you make your formulation in any volume you wish, whether ounces, tablespoons, cups, liters, or grams for example. This is a traditional way to formulate with herbs.

> **Extract Alcohol Percentages**
> A good way to decide how much alcohol to use is this
> **35-40%** for leaves and flowers
> **40-60%** for barks, roots and seeds
> **90%** for Kava Root, Kava is best fat extracted.

Always store your extracts in glass, in a dry, dark spot.

Example- 40% alcohol is 80 proof. All of the alcohol percentages are just baselines, you may find some things work better for you in different ways, please find the way that works best for you.

Then the liquid is poured through a cloth, such as layers of cheesecloth, a kitchen towel with a loose weave or very fine sieve or colander. The herbs that remain are squeezed thoroughly to remove as much of the fluid from them as possible. Extracts can be made of single herbs, or herbal blends, depending upon your needs. Some herbalist run the extracted herbs through a juicer and strain to achieve the best extract they can, or press the extract to get all they can from it. These are all fine ways of doing it, it really is a matter of preference.

It is time-honored traditional magic to begin your extracts on the eve of the new moon, and strain on the full moon, so that the waxing powers of the moon extract the greatest amount of therapeutic agents from the herbs.

Tinctures

A tincture is a diluted extract, traditionally. The tincture is diluted 5x, from the original extract. Unfortunately the term tincture is often misused to describe and extract, so your product would then be weaker. In many cases individuals selling extracts call them tinctures because this is the common name for the process.

In other instances you want a lower percentage solution and a tincture may be exactly what you need.

Glycerin Herbal Extracts

Glycerin is very sweet and will dissolve mucilage, vitamins and minerals. It does not dissolve the resinous or oily properties of herbs very well, such as Myrrh (Commiphora myrrha) Gum. Glycerin is great for extracting bio-flavonoids.

Glycerin is very sweet so it makes an excellent choice for children's remedies, especially when the children are very young and reticent. Glycerin Extracts should be made in small batches because they have a short shelf life about 1 to 3 years, compared to alcohol extracts. Use only pure vegetable glycerin.

Follow the same basic instructions for making the alcohol extract substituting glycerin for alcohol. To make a glycerin extract you can cover your herbs with 100% glycerin alone or combine 3/4-part glycerin with 1/4 part water. Since water is also a solvent I suggest using dried herbs for your glycerin extracts.

Electuary

An Electuary is a sweet way to administer herbs. You can place the herb is a paste made with peanut butter, Tahini, honey or similar ingredient.

An example would be a teaspoon ground herb mixed with enough peanut butter and honey to form a stiff pill shape and this is your electuary.

Electuaries are great for administering herbs to children or individuals with a sweet tooth. Do not give more than eight a day and each dosage depends on the herb/herbs used and amount.

Mellita

Making a Mellita is great for children and individuals not wanting bitter sensations to take herbs. This is not good of course if you wish the bitter principles to help with digestion. Place one ounce of herbs in 20 oz. of water and boil for 20 minutes, covered. Add one ounce of honey and use. Store in glass bottle in the refrigerator for a few months.

Mellita Recipe

Add a half-pound of rose hips to boiling water. Simmer for 15-20 minutes. Allow the mixture to cool and strain through cheesecloth to keep any of the seeds out. Add honey (approximately ½ of the liquid amount to ¾ gauge on thickness, you want it to still be somewhat water and not as thick as a syrup) to the mixture and boil for 3-5 minutes.

Oxymel

An oxymel is an herbal delivery system made from herbs, honey and vinegar. Oxymels are becoming more popular, after waning in popularity for a time.

How to make an Oxymel
Cold Method

Fill a small jar about half to three-fourths full of fresh herbs, chopped. Pour honey over the plants and then the vinegar, organic apple cider vinegar.

You can use 1/3 honey and the rest vinegar or a 50/50 combination. Stir it all together, it may not easily blend, it will with time. Just stir or shake it every day for about two weeks, then strain well. Bottle into a clean jar. Store, bottle it up and store in a cool place or the refrigerator. Use the highest quality honey you can find. Sustainable and local is really important.

Hot Method

Simmer the vinegar and add the herbs, simmer together for twenty minutes. Strain out and stir in honey while the vinegar is still warm. Bottle into a clean jar. Store, bottle it up and store in a cool place or the refrigerator.

Take oxymels by the spoonful when working with a sore throat, thick congested cough or as a general treatment to combat cold symptoms.

Poultice

A poultice is similar to a compress except that plant parts are used rather than liquid extraction. Mash or crush fresh plant parts. Heat them in a pot over boiling water or mix them with a diminutive amount of boiling water. Apply the pulp directly to the skin, as hot as can be tolerated, holding it in place with a gauze bandage. When using dried herb, first powder it and make a paste with 1 tablespoon of powdered herb and a little boiling water or hot cider vinegar, organic. If the paste is likely to irritate the skin, apply it between two layers of cloth. I suggest wool. I secondly suggest fresh wool that has been gently cleaned and is still full of Lanolin. I have a few bags around at all times so I can use the wool I want. Some is barely washed and other pieces are really clean, it depends on what I am, treating with a poultice. Poultices are generally more active than compresses. They are used to arouse circulation, appease aches and pains or draw impurities out through the skin, depending on the herb chosen.

A hot water bottle held against the poultice may keep the heat in for as long as needed. Once it cools, it should be changed and another, as hot as tolerable, applied in its place. Please make sure you don't burn anyone or yourself. Also remember to change the poultice whenever it cools.

Another way to make a Poultice
Simmer enough herbs to cover the affected area for 2 minutes. Squeeze out any excess liquid; rub a little oil on to the affected area to prevent sticking and apply the herb while hot (but not so hot as to burn the skin). Bandage the herb securely in place using gauze or cotton strips. Leave on for up to 3 hours, as required. A wrapping in wool will keep the poultice warm longer.
Application: Apply a new poultice every 2 to 3 hours. Repeat as often as required.

Other types of poultice making
Poultices and Plasters too are used to help draw out toxins and or assist in breathing so their need is to remain in place for long hours. This becomes the main reasons to use these techniques. For the plaster technique, some herbs if left on the skin directly may irritate and cause redness. This action would make your salve or ointment useless.

Poultice, Pulped
Place a quantity of fresh plant material on a clean white cloth. Fold so plant material is inside. Crush with a rolling pin or heavy bottle.
Crushing the herbs directly into the cloth retains all the juices, thus improving

the efficiency of the poultice. Apply to the affected area and over wrap with a cover to hold in body heat.

Poultice, Steamed

Place a colander over a pot of rapidly boiling water. Make sure that the water will not touch the herb material that is placed in the colander. Steam the herbs to wilt. Remove and wait about 10 min then take the steamed herbal mass to the affected area. Cover to hold in the heat. When the poultice cools, reapply as needed.

Plaster

Prepare the herb parts as for either a steamed or pulped poultice, but place the warm mass of pulverized herbs between two layers of cloth before applying to the desired area. Depending on the herbs used, plasters can be left in place for an extended period of time, even overnight.

Fomentation

A fomentation may be used to treat swellings, pain, colds, and flu. Soak a soft white towel or cloth in the desired hot tea infusion. Leave the towel wet but not dripping. Apply the fomentation as hot as the patient can tolerate. To hold in the heat, cover the tea-soaked towel with warm piece of flannel, or even another towel. Repeat and reapply as needed.

I keep a few cloth diapers around just for this reason. They are thick and absorbent.

Microwaves are great for making things warm but you can use a low heat oven, just be careful of gas burning stoves, they could catch fire. Some people hate that I even use the word microwave in an herbal book, but the reality is that many people have them and in a pinch they can be an effective tool. Like all things pros and cons exist.

Cabbage Poultice

Improves lymph drainage and are helpful in removing toxins. Finely chop green cabbage sufficient for the area to be treated.

Place the cabbage in a blender with just enough water to make a thick paste.

Spread the cabbage paste 1" thick over a piece of cheesecloth, muslin or a clean tea towel. The size should be sufficient to cover the preferred part of the body.

Place the cloth, cabbage side onto the skin, over the area to be treated.

Cover with a clean, dry cloth then wrap the whole area in a thick towel or wool flannel cloth.

Leave the cabbage poultice in place for 15 to 60 minutes depending on the rigorousness of the condition and the reactions of the person. It is intended that the treated area should get red and warm but no burning should be allowed to occur. If the person becomes uncomfortable then remove the poultice and wash the area with cool water.

Have the person lie down and rest for the duration of the application.
After removing the poultice wash the area with lukewarm water. The cabbage poultice can be repeated two or three times daily as needed, using fresh cabbage each time.

Compress

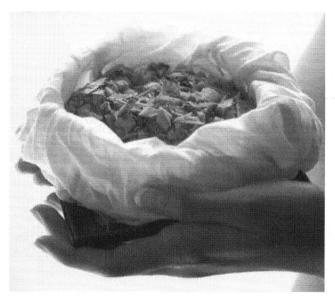

A compress is made by soaking a piece of clean cloth (such as linen, cotton, or gauze) in a decoction or infusion and applying it as hot as can be tolerated to the affected area. When the compress has cooled, it can be soaked again in the reheated liquid and reapplied until the condition has been relieved. Compresses can also be applied cold. I make cold ones for my son's boo-boos. One of my favorite compresses is one that contains Arnica (Arnica montana) and Plantain (Plantago major) for bruising. My sweet sons are extremely rambunctious and I find this one is used an awful lot. I have also made compresses from extracts in water. I find these not only work extremely well but they are easy to use on the go.

Alternate instructions
Wash your hands thoroughly and soak a soft cloth or clean flannel in the liquid mixture, which consists of 2 cups (500 ml) infusion or decoction, or 1 ½

Tablespoon (25 ml) tincture in 2 cups (500 ml) water. Wring out the excess liquid. Before applying, rub a little oil on the affected area to prevent sticking. Place the compress against the affected area. For pain and swellings, secure the compress with plastic film and safety pins and leave for up to 1 to 2 hours. Re-apply as required. You can also layer wool in the plastic to keep the compress warm.

You can also make a compress from essential oil, water and a cloth. Soak a cloth in a bowl of water with a few drops of essential oil, such as Tea Tree (Melaleuca alternifolia) or Lavender (Lavandula angustifolia).

Salve

A salve is a firm beeswax and oil combination that is for external application. Salves can be applied by smoothing on your skin, it will gently spread and melt into the surface of your skin. Salves can be for emotion and physical issues.

Simple Salve Instructions

You need an oil, olive oil or infused oil such as Plantain (Plantago major), Comfrey (Symphytum officinale) or Calendula (Calendula officinalis).

You can estimate the proportions based on the following equivalents.
One pint of oil will need about 1 1/2 ounces of beeswax, or one ounce of oil will need about 1/2 teaspoon of beeswax. There are about 5 teaspoons of beeswax in an ounce.

You then need to heat the oil with the beeswax and mix until all of the wax is melted. Then you add your herbs and essential oils and pour into containers. If the salve is to hard re-melt and add more oil, and if too soft re-melt and add more wax. Instead of wax you can use a vegetarian wax or coconut oil.

Inhalation

An inhalation is when one uses steam to administer herbs or essential oils. The person inhales the steam into their lungs and nose and mouth. This method is great for head colds and sinus ailments.

Inhalation (Portable method)

1 or 2 oz. Bottle or vial
Few grains of large rock salt.
Few drops essential oil.
For clearing nasal passage you could use Rosemary (Rosmarinus officinalis), Eucalyptus, or Peppermint.
For calming oneself you can use Lavender (Lavandula angustifolia), Clary Sage,

for a mild uplifting stimulation is Sweet Orange (Citrus sinensis), Grapefruit (Citrus paradisi) or Mandarin Essential oil.

Over The Bowl Inhalation

Pour boiling water/ very hot water into a bowl. Add a drop or two of essential oil or a few tablespoons of herbs. Then place a towel over your head and bowl and inhale the steam. Please remember not to get your face to close to the hot steam and please be careful not to knock over your bowl.

In the Shower Inhalation

Plug up the tub and start your shower, when a small amount of water has collected add your essential oil and shower. The water will activate the essential oil and provide for inhalation.

Kerchief Inhalation

One can add a few drops to their Kerchief and smell the kerchief when one needs a pick me up.

You can also inhale herbs using a humidifier or vaporizer by adding a few drops to the water. Or you can place a pot of water on the stove add water and herb or essential oil and allow the water to simmer. This is great for children because it is portable and extremely simple to use.

Storing Herbs

Storage containers should be airtight, and dark.
Ideally herbs should be stored in sterilized, dark glass containers with airtight lids.

Label containers

Label all containers with the name of the herb and the date. Glass is the best containers to use. Many restaurants love to donate large glass jars. Many jars can be reused like large pickle, relish, maraschino cherry, etc... Labeling is extremely important, a lot of plants can look and smell alike dry and be complete opposites for healing.
Make sure you also label using the scientific name and the date the herb wash put into the container.

Temperature & Humidity

Store dry herbs at room temperature.

Store in a cool, dry place away from sunlight, moisture, and dust. This is really important.

Shelf life
Leaves, flowers, roots, and other herb parts
Keep for about a year after harvesting in cool place. Store in sterilized, dark glass containers with airtight lids. (May also store in new brown paper bags, which must be kept dry and away from light.) Paper bags inside of Tupperware like containers also work.

Frozen herbs
Herbs frozen in freezer bags keep up to 6 months. You can do this with a lot of your cooking herbs and take out pieces when you want and it tastes like you used fresh herb.

Infusions
Make fresh daily. Store in refrigerator or cool place. They will last a day or two. You can also make in Popsicles for easy child application.

Decoctions
Consume within 48 hours. Store in refrigerator or cool place. You can also make in Popsicles for easy child application.

Tinctures, syrups, and essential oils
Keep for several months or years. Store in dark glass bottles in a cool environment away from sunlight. Store syrup in the refrigerator for up to 1 month, unless a preservative is present such as glycerin or alcohol. Essential oils will evaporate; you must keep them tightly sealed.

Ointments, salves creams, and capsules – These can keep for several months. Store in dark glass jars. You can use hard plastic containers, but they can sometimes degrade, so please use high quality plastic. You can extend the life of creams or anything that combines oil and water by storing them in the refrigerator.

Capsules should be stored as soon as they are made, so they can enter storage in the freshest manner. Anytime left out in the open air will aid in them degrading.

Ointments should be stored in airtight jars and pots. Because they often have a large amount of essential oil, make sure the pots are airtight.

Remedies	Shelf Life
Dried herb material properly stored	1 year
Frozen herbal material	6 months
Infusions and Decoction- refrigerated	48 hours
Extracts/Tinctures properly stored	1-20 years
Glycerides, Oxymels	3-6 months
Essential Oils	1-10 years
Ointments, Salves, Balms	6 month- 2 years
Creams and Lotions, anything with a combination of fat and water.	3-6 months
Capsules	3-6 months

Guidelines for Using Herbs Safely

Here are some rules of thumb for how and when to safely take herbal medicines. Always check with a qualified health practitioner before taking an herbal supplement.

1. Buy organically grown herbs.

2. Discontinue taking any herb immediately if you feel it disagrees with you (you could be allergic to a medicinal herb just as you could a drug). Even if you know you don't like something but you can't find why you don't like it, discontinue use, your body is trying to tell you something. Listen to your body.

3. Be certain the herb has been properly identified as the herb you think it is. This is especially important for using bulk herbs. LABEL!

4. Pay close attention to recommended dosages for different herbs and properly adjust dosages for children, elders and those with weak constitutions.

5. Many herbal teas and herbs in food are safe for daily use over time, but stronger forms of herbs including extracts should not be used for more than brief periods without a naturopathic doctor or trained herbalist's supervision. Some herbs cannot be used under certain circumstances. Learn about your body and your health.

6. If you have a chronic medical condition, use herbs under medical supervision. Some herbs will interact with medication and they should not be used without the proper education and supervision.

Recipe Lingo!

As you are reading through the recipes you may find familiar and unfamiliar terms. So we are explaining them briefly, hopefully this will make the recipe easier to follow.

tsp- is a teaspoon

TBSP., tbsp. - is a tablespoon

oz. is an abbreviation for an ounce

eo, EO- Essential Oil

c- is a cup

Drop- a drop is literally a drop, from a 2 oz. sized dropper. These can be bought individually or as part of a bottle set. You can also use a similar sized pipette or in a pinch a cocktail straw as you would a pipette.

Part- Very simply a part is 1 of something. Depending on the recipe it can be 1 teaspoon, 1 tablespoon or 1 cup. A part is a consistent part of the recipe. So for example:

2 parts Red Raspberry (Rubus ideaeus) Leaf

1 parts Nettles (Urtica dioica)

Equivalency Measurements
1 pinch = less than 1/8 teaspoon (dry)
1 dash = 3 drops to 1/4 teaspoon (liquid)
3 teaspoons = 1 tablespoon = 1/2 ounce (liquid and dry)
2 tablespoons = 1 ounce (liquid and dry)
4 tablespoons = 2 ounces (dry and liquid) = 1/4 cup
1 cup = 8 ounces (liquid) = 1/2 pint
16 cups = 128 ounces (liquid) = 4 quarts = 1 gallon
Approximate Equivalents
1 quart (liquid) = close to 1 liter
8 tablespoons = 4 ounces = 1/2 cup = 1 stick butter

This would be a simple pregnancy tea recipe. If you are making 1 cup then a teaspoon of each herb would be enough. If you were blending it in bulk you could use 2 parts Red Raspberry Leaf (each part being 2 cups, making a total of 4 cups) and 1part Nettle leaf (the part being 2 cups, so 2 cups would be added). You would add this to a large mixing bowl and mix until it is fully incorporated. You would then either package or place into a dry container for storage.

2 EVERYTHING OIL

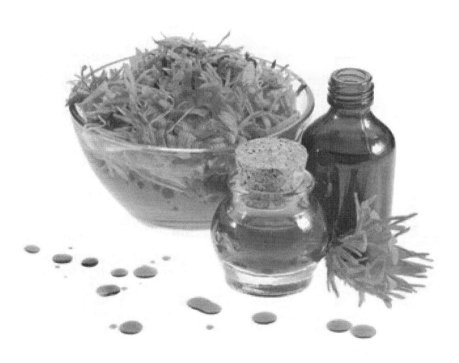

Madlen/Shutterstock

Infused Oils

Infused oils are often used topically for skin issues, or internally as a flavoring for food. An infused oil is also called a medicinal oil or herbal oil. They can be used as part of another product like a salve, balm or lotion or on their own as a massage oil or liniment.

Infused oil instructions

Medicinal Oils can be used alone as a massage oil, medicinal application, salad oil or dipping oil, these are all forms of infused oils. Additionally they can also be used as medicine in the form of salves, balms, liniment oils, and lotions.

The quality of an infused oil depends on a few things. The quality of the herbs in the infused oil. Are the herbs clean, fresh, and relieved of excessive moisture?

The quality of the oil used, cold processed, expeller pressed, organic, etc... The oil should smell like what it comes from, sunflower seeds for sunflower oil, olives for olive oil, and so on. The oil part is often called a carrier oil in recipes.

Fresh versus dried herbs. In my opinion in almost all circumstances used fresh herb is far better than using dried herbs for infused oils.

Time, quality, purity and cleanliness are all essential to a good infused oil.

Bulk freshly picked herb. Depending on the amount you will be making between 1 cup and a pound. You essentially want enough to fill your contains almost to the top.

Clean Sterile Jars

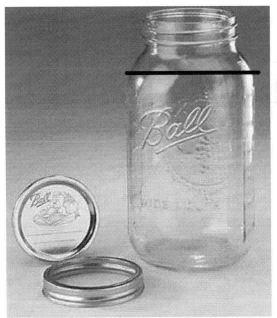

Maximum fill line. Always use a clean sterile jar.

Oil- Cold Pressed and Expeller pressed oils are both all natural and involve no chemicals. Then you have traditional oils that are extracted usually in a combination. Cold Pressed and Expeller oils are often preferred because they essentially squeeze or press the oils out, they can also be expensive. Use the highest quality oil you can afford. For the sake of price you will find sunflower, safflower and olive the most cost effective. You can even find organic and oils originating from the US in most grocery and box stores now.

Make sure no matter what you use that you use the highest quality oil and you know its origin, and Latin name for labeling. Even if you are making items just for friends you want to have everything properly labeled in case of reaction.

The method I like to use most for infusing oils is this, use a clean sterile jar, and fill until the maximum filled line, as pictured on the previous page. Cover the herb with oil. Allow the oils to be absorbed by the plants cellular walls for a few hours. After the herb has absorbed some of the oil, add more if needed. What you want is for the oil to completely cover the plant matter, leaving no room for air, moisture and potential contamination.

You also need to do some preparation with the plant matter beforehand. When you harvest the plant matter make sure it is clean. I use flour sack towels and brush all of the excess dirt and moisture off. Make sure when you harvest it is after the morning dew has evaporated, at least a day after the last rain and that the evening dew has not set. In addition you will need to lie the plant matter out on a tea towel or paper towel for at least 3 hours to absorb any released moisture, if the season has been especially wet, leave the plants to wilt overnight, this allows the release of excess water and prevents potential spoilage.

Solar infusion: One you have gotten the herb ready for infusion do the following. Place in a warm, sunny window and let infuse for about 2 weeks. Strain and rebottle. If you would like to increase the strength of the oil you can add fresh plant material and allow infusion for two more weeks.

Oven Extraction: Place the herbs and oil in a canning jar, or a container with a tight fitting lid. Put them in a pan with enough water to cover the bottom half of the jar. I like using a casserole dish. Turn the oven on the lowermost temperature possible and heat for several hours. If you have a warming oven you can use this.

Double boiler method: Place herbs and oil in a double boiler, covered with a tightly fitting lid and bring to a slow simmer. Slowly allow it to heat, on low heat for 1/2 hour to an hour, do not overheat under any circumstances that will ruin your oil. The lower the heat and longer the infusion time the better quality of oil. This can also be done on top of a woodstove.

Crockpot method or electric roaster method: Add as much oil as you want and plant matter. Set on the lowest heat possible, and allow to the oil to warm for a few hours at least. Electric roasters have an even lower heat source and herbal oils can be left too steep for 2 weeks. Make sure the temperature is less than 120-130 degrees F. You can use a candy thermometer to monitor temperature.

Once the herbs have been infused into the oil use cheesecloth to strain the oil and gently press, then strain the mixture again. The re-bottle the oil in clean sterile jars, properly label and store in a clean, dry, dark place, such as a cabinet, pantry, etc...

Making Infused Oils Tips
1. Pick the plant on a dry, sunny day. After any morning dew has evaporated. This is really important, any plant matter with excessive moisture can promote mold and bacteria growth.
2. Do not use any diseased or soiled parts. Do not wash any part of the plant, the plant is dirty scrub it off with a stiff dry brush, toothbrush or a dry washcloth. Some roots that are really dirty can also be peeled if needed.
3. Chop or rip the plant coarsely.
4. Completely fill a clean, very dry jar with the chopped herb, to the fill line.
5. Slowly pour oil into the jar, poke the plant material down with a butter knife or chopstick to compact the material loosely and release any additional air. Cover all material with the oil. After the oil has sat and absorbed for a few hours add oil to the lid level.
6. Make sure the oil is properly lidded or corked.
7. Store at cool room temperature or refrigerate.
8. Proper Labels for Oil need to contain a name if you want one, the ingredients, this includes the herbs common name and the Latin or scientific name, and what type of oil is used, Latin and common name also. These label guidelines really should be used for all herbal remedies and skin care items. Proper labeling will make sure you know what is in each container, the user knows and having all of the ingredients will assist if an issue occurs.
9. Date your items. Make sure you put the made date on each item.

Trouble Shooting Infused Oil Issues

Mold can really be an issue if your oils are not properly done. Do not despair we all have had an issue with an oil molding.

If you do not fill the jar with oil completely to the top, mold will grow in the air space left. To save your preparation, completely remove the mold and fill the jar to the top with fresh oil.

The jar needs to be completely dry. If not mold will grow. You can dry your jars for five minutes immediately prior to use prevent this problem. Some people like to blast the jar with a hair drier just to be sure, that can prove beneficial on really humid days.

If the jar is put in the sun or left near a heat source, the plant material as the cells become infused with oil will cause condensation and push the water from the cell walls, this provides the moisture necessary for colonies of mold. If this occurs remove the mold and pour oil and plant material into a fresh jar to save this.

If any of the plant material was damp or wet when combined with the oil, mold will grow throughout the oil. Saving it is impossible, dump the oil and start again. Wilt your plant material overnight, or in the over on low for 1-2 hours. Make sure you do not bake the herbs, they should still be pliable, and not crispy feeling. If you use dried herb material this will not be an issue, but a lot of herbs respond better to oil infusion when fresh.

Infusion Herbs

You can use all kinds of herbs for infused oils. Here are some commonly used herbs to make infused oils and what they are good for. Some of these recipes call for essential oils, a good rule of thumb is to add the essential oils (EO) after the oil is strained and bottled, and add no more than 20 drops per ounce, I tend to advise adding less at first, then a few more drops as needed.

Essential oils are a concentrated hydrophobic (repels water) liquid comprising of the volatile aroma compounds from plants. Essential oils are also recognized as volatile oils. An oil is "essential" in the sense that it carries a distinctive scent, or essence, of the plant. Essential oils are usually extracted by the process of distillation. Steam distillation is often the primary method used. Other processes include expression or solvent extraction. Essential oils are used in cosmetics, medicinal products, perfumes, soaps and other products, and for adding scents to incense and household cleaning products.

Carrier Oils are nut, seed, fruit and vegetable oils used in herbal and aromatherapy products. They have healing properties of their own.

Carrier oils also known as or called base oils. Essentially they are vegetable or nut oils that are used to dilute essential oils, CO2s and absolutes before applying to the skin. They "carry" the essential oil onto the skin. Different carrier oils offer

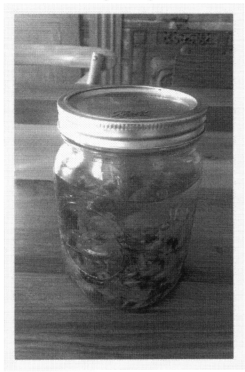

different properties and the choice of carrier oil can depend on the therapeutic benefit being sought.

Carrier oils are generally cold-pressed vegetable oils derived from the fatty portions of the plant. Unlike essential oils that evaporate and have a concentrated aroma, carrier oils do not evaporate or impart their aroma as strongly as essential oils.

Examples of carrier oils are sweet almond, apricot kernel, grapeseed, avocado, peanut, olive, pecan, macadamia nut, sesame, evening primrose, walnut and wheat germ.

Commonly Infused Herbs
Arnica flowers (Arnica montana) - This is an external and topical treatment for physical pain, sprains, bruising and other injuries. Use immediately after vigorous exertion, an injury or to prevent, relieve and reduce swelling, bruising and pain. Arnica should not be used internally.

Borage-(Borago officinalis) - A prized oil for its abundant dietary, health, cosmetic and medicinal benefits. Infuse the flowers and the leaves.

Calendula-(Calendula officinalis)- This oil is the most successful oil for assisting with dry, sensitive and damaged skin, skin inflammations, rashes, diaper irritations, and other skin issues. Makes a wonderful baby's oil and is exceptional for those with sensitive skin.

Chickweed-(Stellar media)- Best known in its use for treating pruritus and itchy skin, it is also used to treat: eczema; acne; ulcers; hemorrhoids, varicose veins, psoriasis, inflammation, vaginitis, urticaria, contact rashes, boils; wounds; abscesses, skin allergies, and other skin problems.

Comfrey-(Symphytum officinale.) Traditionally used for general wound healing, treatment of bruises and for skin cell proliferation. Not to be used on dirty or open wounds.

St. John's Wort (Hypericum perforatum) A valuable anti-inflammatory which can help speed the healing of wounds, bruises, varicose veins, sunburns, bee stings, and mild burns. Frequently used as a breast massage oil especially after radiation treatments. Personally this is one for my favorite oils. I think it feels like sunshine on my skin. The picture is the beginning of a St. John's Wort oil infusion, using olive oil and fresh St. John's Wort flowers.

Mullein Flower (Verbascum thapsus) has antiviral, antifungal, and antibacterial properties and is an age old remedy for ear infections.

Garlic Oil- This is a popular remedy for earaches, and great on salads.

Massage Oils

Massage oils are made from carrier oils and essential oils. You can used infused oils, plain carrier oil or butters to make massage oil. Massage oil facilitates massage by lubricating the friction between the skin and the hand allowing for smooth massages. Massage oil also nourishes and moisturizes skin. All massage oils need to be stored in dry bottles, glass works well, make sure the bottles are clean and dry. Store massage oils in a clean dry place, like a cupboard.

Some of these massage oil recipes will be for relaxation and the overall scent, others are for therapeutic use. The therapeutic use of massage oils is rooted in ancient history. Massage has always been considered one of the basic considerations of care, touch. Massage is giving and receiving healing touch.

Oils For Athletes
Massage Oil for Athletes
10 drops Eucalyptus (Eucalyptus globulus) Essential Oil
10 drops Rosemary (Rosmarinus officinalis) Essential Oil
10 drops Thyme (Thymus vulgaris) Essential Oil
2 tablespoons Carrier oil
 Combine oils and store in airtight glass container. Before jogging or running, rub the oil over your feet, ankles, calves, thighs, buttocks, lower back, and arms. The Thyme can assist in soothing sprains. Eucalyptus can help to reduce inflammation and pain. Rosemary (Rosmarinus officinalis) can assist in healing muscular sprains.

Leg Cramp Oil
This oil is so soothing and relaxing on tired muscles. It is not only great for leg

cramps, but also for varicose veins, varicosities and sore backs. Put the following ingredients into a container and shake well before using:

2 ounces St. John's Wort (Hypericum perforatum) infused oil

5 drops   Neroli (Citrus aurantium) essential oil

5 drops Grapefruit (Citrus paradisi) essential oil

Apply in a gentle upward motions.

Sore Muscle Oil

1 part Peppermint (Mentha piperita)

1 part St. John's Wort (Hypericum perforatum)

1 part Arnica (Arnica montana) flower

This is great for sore muscles and aches and pains associated with exercise and over exertion.

Super Sore Muscle Oil

1 part Arnica (Arnica montana) flower

1 part Peppermint (Mentha piperita) Leaf

1 part Valerian (Valeriana officinalis, Valerianaceae) Root

A few drops of Peppermint essential oil, not to exceed 10 drops per ounce of completed oil. The essential oil is added when the oil is completed and re-bottled. Many oils are also great on foods, and good medicine like Basil (Ocimum basilicum) Garlic, Oregano (Oreganum vulgare), Lemon Balm (Melissa officinalis), Cinnamon (Cinnamomum verum), etc...

You can have a lot of fun making seasoned oils.

Knee Oil

1 cup infused St. John's Wort (Hypericum perforatum) Oil

10 drops Peppermint (Mentha piperita) EO

10 drops Black Pepper (Piper unigram) EO

10 drops Lavender (Lavandula angustifolia) EO

Combine well and apply liberally to the affected area.

Tennis Elbow Oil

½ cup Arnica (Arnica montana) Infused Oil

½ cup St. John's Wort (Hypericum perforatum) Oil

20 drops Eucalyptus globulus EO

10 drops Ginger (Zingiber officinale) EO

10 drops Helichrysum (Helichrysum angustifolia) EO

Combine well and apply liberally to the affected area.
I find that massaging firmly into the area really helps.

Massage Oil for Tendonitis
10 drops Rosemary (Rosmarinus officinalis) Essential Oil
10 drops Eucalyptus (Eucalyptus globulus) Essential Oil
10 drops Peppermint (Mentha piperita) Essential Oil
2 Tbs. Carrier Oil such as sweet almond oil, or apricot kernel oil
Combine oils and store in airtight glass container. Use as a cool massage oil for affected hands, wrists, and joint after cool compresses.

Acute Pain- For Joint Pain
2 oz. carrier oil or infused Chickweed oil
10 drops Juniper (Juniperus communis) EO
1 drop Pine (Pinus sylvestris) EO
2 drops Rosemary (Rosmarinus officinalis) EO
Apply to affected joint.

Massage Oil for Shin Splints
To ¼ cup carrier oil or infused Chickweed oil add
6 drops Lemon (Citrus limon) EO
4 drops Cypress (Cupressus sempervirens) EO
5 drops Lavender (Lavendula officinalis) EO
Mix well and use on shins, and other affected areas. Ice packs and elevating the legs also helps.

Massage Oil for Chilblains
1 cup Chickweed infused oil
30 drops Lavender (Lavandula angustifolia) and 30 drops Rosemary (Rosmarinus officinalis) EO
Apply to affected areas.

Massage Oil- Acute Inflammation
5 drops Chamomile (Matricaria chamomilla) EO
3 drops Helichrysum (Helichrysum angustifolia) EO
1 drop Myrrh (Commiphora myrrha) EO
2 tablespoons carrier oil
Massage into inflamed areas.

Arthritis Oils
Arthritis Massage Oil
4 oz. Carrier oil such as sweet almond oil, or apricot kernel oil
10 drops Black Pepper (Piper nigrum) EO
10 drops Fennel (Foeniculum vulgare) EO
10 drops Juniper (Juniperus communis) EO
10 drops Peppermint (Mentha piperita) EO
Massage on the affected area. If too strong add more carrier oil. If not potent enough add a few more drops of one of the oils. This works wonderfully on sore joints and arthritic spots on the body.

Arthritis Blend
2 ounces carrier oil such as sweet almond oil, or apricot kernel oil.
20 drops Roman Chamomile (Matricaria chamomilla) EO
5 drops Black Pepper (Piper nigrum) EO
Massage the affected area. Great on tissues surrounding the effected joints.

Arthritis Blend II
2 ounces carrier oil such as sweet almond oil, or apricot kernel oil
10 drops Atlas Cedarwood (Cedrus atlantica) wood EO
5 drops Black Pepper (Piper nigrum) EO
5 drops Rosemary (Rosmarinus officinalis) EO
Massage into the affected area.

Back Pain Blends
Back Ache Massage Oil
2 oz. St. John's Wort (Hypericum perforatum) infused oil.
10 drops Peppermint (Mentha piperita) EO
5 drops Juniper (Juniperus communis) EO
2 drops Lavender (Lavendula officinalis) EO
This is wonderful when used on the lower back.
Massage in firmly, into the sacrum, lower back and upper buttocks.

Lower Back Pain
½ cup Arnica (Arnica montana) infused oil
½ cup St. John's Wort (Hypericum perforatum) infused oil
20 drops Clary Sage (Salvia sclarea)EO

20 drops Lavender (Lavandula angustifolia) EO
10 drops Chamomile EO
Apply to the lower back region.

Lower Back Pain II
½ cup Arnica (Arnica montana) infused oil
½ cup St. John's Wort (Hypericum perforatum) infused oil
20 drops Rosemary (Rosmarinus officinalis) EO
10 drops Yarrow (Achillea millefolium) EO
10 drops Frankincense EO
Apply to the lower back region.

Sciatica
1 part St. John's Wort (Hypericum perforatum) flower
1 part Arnica (Arnica montana) flower
Arnica will relax and soothe the muscles that are surrounding the nerve and St. John's Wort soothes the nerve.

Nerve Pain Oil
10 drops German Chamomile EO
6 drops Marjoram EO
6 drops Helichrysum (Helichrysum angustifolia) EO
10 drops Lavender (Lavandula angustifolia) EO
2 ounces infused St. John's Wort (Hypericum perforatum) oil
1 ounce Plantain (Plantago major) infused oil
Combine well and apply liberally to the affected area.

Massage Oil- Lumbar Pain
2 tablespoons carrier oil
10 drops Rosemary (Rosmarinus officinalis) EO
10 drops Marjoram (Origanum majorana) EO
10 drops Sage (Salvia officinalis) EO
Or
10 drops Lavender (Lavendula officinalis) EO
10 drops Eucalyptus (Eucalyptus globulus) EO
10 drops Basil (Ocimum basilicum) EO
Place the massage oil on the lumbar region.

Circulation
Circulation Massage Oil
½ cup Sweet Almond Oil
10 drops of the following Nutmeg (Myristica fragrans), Orange (Citrus sinensis) and Lemon (Citrus limon) EO
1-2 drops Cinnamon EO
Apply lightly to the affected area.

Circulation Oil 2
½ cup St. John's Wort (Hypericum perforatum) oil, infused oil
10 drops Neroli (Citrus aurantium) EO
5 drops Bay EO
Apply to the affected area. This feels lovely applied in long strokes on tired or swollen legs. I like it after a long flight.

Vein Oil
This is helpful with Varicose Veins. Originally made this recipe in 1998, when I opened my herbal company. I was surprised at how well it sold, word of mouth alone.
10 drops Palmarosa EO
8 drops Cypress EO
10 drops Grapefruit (Citrus paradisi) EO
7 drops German Chamomile EO
1 ounce St. John's Wort infused oil
Combine ingredients. Apply externally directly over problem area (as described above) one or two times a day.

Colds and Flu
Massage Oil for Common Colds
2 drops Lemon (Citrus limon) EO
2 drops Eucalyptus (Eucalyptus globulus) EO
2 drops Rosemary (Rosmarinus officinalis) EO
1 teaspoon Carrier Oil
Combine oils and store in tightly covered glass jar.
Massage around the chest, neck, and sinus area with the oil.

Massage Oil for Dry Cough
3 drops Eucalyptus (Eucalyptus globulus) EO

2 drops Thyme (Thymus vulgaris) EO
1 teaspoon Carrier Oil
Combine oils and store in airtight glass container. Use oil mixture to massage over the back and chest.

Massage Oil for the Flu

2 drops Tea Tree (Melaleuca alternifolia) EO
3 drops Eucalyptus (Eucalyptus globulus) EO
1 teaspoon Carrier Oil
Combine oils and use for a full body massage. Then go to bed.

Ear Infection Oil
Massage Oil for Ear Infections

3 drops Tea Tree (Melaleuca alternifolia) Essential Oil
1 drop Thyme (Thymus vulgaris) Essential Oil
2 drops Lavender (Lavendula officinalis) Essential Oil
1 teaspoon Carrier Oil
Combine oils and store in airtight container. Massage gently with oil mixture around the ear area, up the neck, and across the cheekbone.

Foot Massage Oil
Massage Oil for Feet

5 drops Lavender (Lavendula officinalis) Essential Oil
3 drops Thyme (Thymus vulgaris) Essential Oil
4 drops Peppermint (Mentha piperita) Essential Oil
  Combine oils. Use 5 drops of oil mixture to 2 teaspoons carrier oil for each foot. Massage feet with this blend before and after athletic activity.

Massage Oil for Feet 2

5 drops Rosemary (Rosmarinus officinalis) Essential Oil
3 drops Peppermint (Mentha piperita) Essential Oil
4 drops Lavender (Lavendula officinalis) Essential Oil
  Combine Essential Oils. Use 5 drops of oil mixture to 2 teaspoons carrier oil for both feet. Massage feet with this blend before and after walking, running, or jogging. This is also great if you're on your feet all day.

Headache
Massage Oil for General Headache
3 drops Lavender (Lavendula officinalis) Essential Oil
1 drop Peppermint (Mentha piperita) Essential Oil
1 drop Vegetable Oil
Combine oils and use to massage around the temples and base of the skull, and along the hair line for headache.

Massage Oil for Gastric Headache
1 drop Rosemary (Rosmarinus officinalis) Essential Oil
2 drops Peppermint (Mentha piperita) Essential Oil
1 drop Lavender (Lavendula officinalis) Essential Oil
Combine oils and use to massage the back of the neck.
Also you can inhale 1 drop of the mixture on a tissue or use 3-5 drops in a steam inhalation.

Herpes
Herpes Helper Oil- Chickenpox, cold sores (do not use near eyes)
2 parts Lemon Balm (Melissa officinalis)
1 part Oregano (Oreganum vulgare)
2 -4 cloves garlic (depending on the jar size).
Add to a jar and cover with olive oil. Allow the oil to infuse for at least 2 weeks, shaking gently once a day. Strain well before use. When applying use a clean cotton swab each time. Dab the affected area with the infused oil.

Shingles Oil
1 cup infused St. John's Wort (Hypericum perforatum) Oil
10 drops St. John's Wort EO (Hypericum perforatum)
10 drops Sandalwood EO (Santalum spicatum)
10 drops Peppermint EO (Mentha piperita)
10 drops Ravensara EO (Agathophyllum aromatica)
Thickly apply to the rash. The rash will be causing immense pain, if you are applying on another person, the best bet is to just do it and both of you grit your teeth. If it is on a person's face, they should apply it themselves.

Indigestion
Massage Oil Indigestion
2 drops Peppermint (Mentha piperita) EO

2 drops Sweet Orange (Citrus sinensis) EO
2 tablespoons carrier oil EO
Massage abdomen lightly.

Massage Oil- Helpful with constipation pain.
12 drops Rosemary (Rosmarinus officinalis) EO
12 drops Lemon (Citrus limon) EO
5 drops Peppermint (Mentha piperita) EO
2 Tbs. Carrier Oil
Combine oils and store in airtight glass container. Use a small amount of oil in the palm of your hand to massage in a clockwise direction over the lower abdomen three times a day. Constipation can have underlying causes. Check dietary habits and hydration. Never rub over areas of acute pain. If abdominal tenderness, rigidity, or distention is noted, consult a medical professional. Always use prudence in abdominal massage, avoiding painful areas to prevent possible complications.

Menopause
Menopause Massage oil
2 tablespoons carrier oil
5 drops Clary Sage (Salvia sclarea)EO
5 drops Jasmine (Jasminum grandiflorum) EO
2 drops Nutmeg (Myristica fragrans) EO
Massage on your body lightly, massage on your shoulders and chest.

Hot Flash Massage oil
2 tablespoons carrier oil
10 drops Jasmine (Jasminum grandiflorum) EO
11 drops Geranium (Pelargonium graveolens) EO
5 drops Lemon (Citrus limon) EO
2 drops Sage (Salvia officinalis) EO
Massage on your body lightly.

Hot Flash- Massage Oil
2 tablespoons carrier oil
10 drops Clary Sage (Salvia sclarea)EO
3 drops Sage Salvia officinalis EO
10 drops Geranium (Pelargonium graveolens) EO

5 drops Lemon (Citrus limon) EO
Massage all over body, lightly.

Menopause- Night and Day Sweats
In 2 tablespoons carrier oil add
12 drops Grapefruit (Citrus paradisi) EO
5 drops Lime (Citrus aurantifolia) EO
5 drops Sweet Orange (Citrus sinensis) EO
2 drops Sage (Salvia officinalis) EO
Massage on your body lightly.

Menstruation
Massage Oil- Menstrual Cramps ¼ cup carrier oil add
6 drops Basil (Ocimum basilicum) EO
4 drops Lemongrass (Cymbopogon citratus) EO
4 drops Marjoram (Origanum majorana) EO
This massage oil is excellent for menstrual cramps. Massage into the uterine area of the stomach

Menstrual Cramp Oil II
6 drops Lavender (Lavendula officinalis) EO
4 drops Marjoram (Origanum majorana) EO
4 drops Chamomile (Matricaria chamomilla) or Clary Sage (Salvia sclarea) EO
4 drops Geranium (Pelargonium graveolens) EO
1-2 drops Ginger (Zingiber officinale) EO
2 ounces carrier oil like Olive oil, Apricot Kernel, or similar oil. Massage over the abdomen and uterine area.

Skin Issue Massage Oils
Lavender Infused Oil This is a great oil for infants, relaxation and skin issues like eczema.
Fill a jar with lavender flower and cover with olive oil.
Prepare and decant as you would an infused oil.

Massage Oil (great for winter itch or nonspecific itching)
4 oz. Carrier oil
10 drops Balsam Peru/Peru Balsam EO (name is commonly interchanged)
5 drops Helichrysum (Helichrysum angustifolia) EO

5 drops Bergamot (Citrus bergamia) EO
This massage oil is good for winter's dry skin.

Dry Skin
1 part Calendula (Calendula officinalis) flower
½ part Chickweed (Stellaria media)
Make as an infused oil, using fresh plant matter. Add the plant matter to a dry jar and cover with olive oil. Allow it too steep for 4-6 weeks. Follow the infused oil instructions. Use on dry skin.

Eczema Oil
1 part Chickweed (Stellaria media) Infused oil
1 part Calendula (Calendula officinalis) flower Infused oil
Apply on affected area.

Severe Eczema Blend
1 part Chickweed (Stellaria media)
1 part Calendula (Calendula officinalis) flower
1 part St. John's Wort (Hypericum perforatum)
Mix the oils together, a part is the amount you want it to be. 1 part can be a teaspoon, tablespoon, ½ cup, cup, etc... Mix in a container before bottling, into clear dry containers.

Scalp
Rosemary Infused Oil
This oil can be really beneficial for scalp issues, like dandruff and itchiness. Slightly warm the oil, and gently rub a small amount into the scalp and/or through the length of the hair, or just the tips if you have damaged ends wrap a towel around your head, and leave on for one hour. Shampoo out.
Fill a quart jar with fresh Rosemary.
Cover with olive, argon or sesame oil.
Prepare and decant as you would an infused oil.

Bhringaraj Oil
Fill a jar with Bhringaraj leaf (Eclipta alba)
Cover with Sesame oil and allow it to infuse for at least 3 weeks.
This oil is traditionally popular with hair issues, and often used to promote restful sleep when massaged into the neck and the shoulders before bed.

Brahmi Oil
Fill a jar with
1 part Brahmi leaf (Centella asiatica)
1 part Bacopa herb (Bacopa monniera)
Cover the herb with warmed coconut oil (1/3) of the oil, and sesame oil (2/3) of the added oil.
Prepare and decant as you would an infused oil. Infuse for at least two weeks, you may need to warm this oil to make it so you can strain it. If I have coconut oil that is setting up a lot, I gently warm it every day, or put it in a sunny window. This oil is good for calming the nervous system.

Pregnancy
Labor Massage Oil
1 part Jasmine (Jasminum grandiflorum) Essential oil (5 drops)
1 part Rose Essential oil
2 parts Geranium (Pelargonium graveolens) Essential oil
½ cup carrier oil
Massage on abdomen only when in active labor.

Labor Massage Oil II
2 oz. Carrier oil
5 drops Rose EO
6 drops Ylang Ylang (Cananga odorata) EO
12 drops Clary Sage (Salvia sclarea) EO
2 drops Sweet Orange (Citrus sinensis) EO
Massage on abdomen only when in active labor. It really helps when the massage follows the path of the contractions.

Pregnancy- Aching Legs
1 oz. carrier oil
15 drops Lavender (Lavendula officinalis) EO
10 drops Rosemary (Rosmarinus officinalis) EO
Use only in Labor. EO
Massage on thighs and calves only when in active labor, or for the postpartum period. If varicose veins are present please do not massage or stoke the vein directly.

Some sources say to avoid Rosemary (Rosmarinus officinalis) essential oil if you suffer epilepsy. But as with everything please look up each oil and herb yourself.

Stretch Mark Massage Oil
1 cup cocoa butter, melted
2 tablespoons flaxseed oil
2 tablespoons rose hip seed oil
3 tablespoons wheat germ oil
1 tablespoon Borage Oil
12 drops Lavender (Lavendula officinalis) EO
10 drops Neroli (Citrus aurantium) EO
6 drops Vetiver (Vetiveria zizanoides) EO
Blend the melted cocoa butter with the other oils. Pour the mixture to a clean jar. Add the essential oils. Allow the mixture to cool to a comfortable temperature before using it. Use this wonderful blend once or twice a day. This is great for pregnant bellies and breasts.

Belly Balm or Stretch Mark Prevention Oil

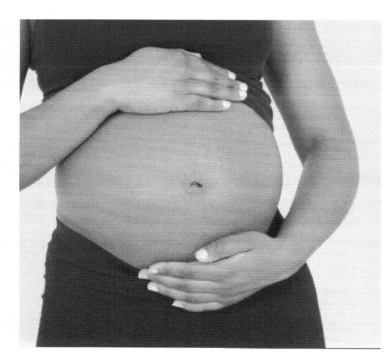

This oil feels wonderful going on. It is smooth and moisturizing and can help with the itching that so often happens when the skin starts stretching. In a double boiler, melt the carrier oils listed below. Carrier oils are nut or seed oils, like almond oil, Shea butter, coconut butter and olive oil, for example. These are pressed and not distilled.

1 cup coconut oil

¼ cup cocoa butter

1/8 cup apricot, almond or grape seed oil

1/8 cup Kukui nut (Aleurites moluccana) oil, Shea butter or mango butter (I love using mango butter.)

When these oils have melted completely, remove the mixture from the heat.

Stir well and add the essential oils, then incorporate them in well.

10–20 drops Sandalwood (Santalum album) (try to purchase from an ethical source*)

15 drops Patchouli (Pogostemon cablin)

15 drops Sweet Orange (Citrus sinensis) essential oil

There are additional options for essential oils. Use what you like and/or can find locally. You can also try rosewood, rose, Lavender (Lavandula angustifolia), tangerine and Neroli (Citrus aurantium). If you blend your own mixture, be sure to keep the amount of essential oils used at less than 50 drops total.

Massage the balm all over thighs, breasts, stomach and anywhere else that needs nourishing and moisturizing. I have also used this on my face. The oil is nourishing to all of you skin, not just skin that is being stretched by pregnancy. This also works on teens who are developing stretch marks from growing so fast.

Infant Care
Infant Massage Oil

¼ cup Apricot Kernel oil

5 drops Lavender (Lavendula officinalis) Essential oil

3 drops Grape seed oil

Massage on infant after baths and when baby's skin is dry.

Cradle Cap blend

In 4 oz. Olive oil infuse Calendula flower and chamomile flower.

Cradle cap is a fact of life. It is when the oily scalp of baby causes a "pile up" of excess skin that becomes flaky and crusty. Do not pick. Apply an oil and gently comb the scalp and hair, use a cotton ball in the eyebrows and behind ears if it is present there. Wash head gently. Use a nice olive oil. Do not use mineral oil.

Or

At night apply the olive oil and allow it to stay on baby's head until morning. Comb out and wash in the morning.

Or

You can slough off the oily scalp and oil with a very soft toothbrush.

Coconut Oil or Butter Infusions

Coconut Oil, or Butters like Shea, Mango, Cocoa Butter, Kukui Nut, Cupuacu, Murumuru are all butters you can purchase.

You may have not heard of the following oils, so here is a little information on them.

Cupuacu Butter gives it the capacity to restore elasticity to the skin and treat skin conditions including eczema and dermatitis

Murumuru Butter is pressed from the reddish-orange fruits of the Astrocaryum murumuru tree. This tall palm tree is native to Brazil and other regions of the Amazon. Great for dry skin, and eczema.

Infused Murumuru Butter for Eczema

Melt down 1 cup Murumuru butter in a double boiler

Add ¼ cup Calendula (Calendula officinalis) flower, cut the heat to low.

After an hour of low heat, remove from heat and allow too steep for 24 hours. Occasionally warm back up.

Add 10 drops of Lavender (Lavandula angustifolia) essential oil, and allow to cool. Use on eczema, dry or tired skin.

You can also make this infused butter with Mango, Shea or Cupuacu butters.

Creams with Infused Oils

Vegan or Not

I've categorized the ingredients into two separate groups, the oils and the waters.

All lotions and creams are emulsifications of water and oil.

Oils 3/4 cup of one of the following

Apricot (a good light oil for oily skin)

Almond (for a rich non-greasy or heavy oil

Olive (great for a rich, thick, wintertime cream)

You can use a blend of the oils as long as 3/4 of a cup is the final measurement. For a dry skin you can infuse Calendula, Plantain (Plantago major), or Chickweed (Stellaria media). For irritated skin you can use St. John's Wort oil.

1/3 cup Coconut Oil

2 Tablespoons Mango Butter or Kokum Butter

These are nut butters from the seeds of these plants.

1/2 ounce Shea Butter, Candelilla Wax, Carnauba Wax or Beeswax- Both waxes are plant source waxes. Shea butter comes from the seeds of the Karite tree and Beeswax is bee derived.

Waters 2/3 cup Distilled Water, you can also use floral waters or infusions. Rose water, lavender and orange water are very popular in lotions. You can get high quality rosewaters at many places, but I often get them at Asian or Indian markets. It is often high quality and food grade.

1/2 cup Aloe Vera

Buy this; sometimes when the Aloe comes from a fresh plant source, the cream can become rancid.

2 Vitamin E Caps or a (r) teaspoon Vitamin E Powder

5-10 drops Essential Oil (optional). You want the essential oil to not be to overpowering, but when you make the lotion/cream for the first time use less essential oil and add up to 5-10 drops, or even more with experience.

Basic Cream Instructions
The next part can be a little tricky

Heat the oils over low heat until the solid oils melt into the liquid oils. Also, warm the water (but not the entire water group). When the water and the oil cool to about the same temperature, add the water and the rest of the water group to your blender. Blend. Next, slowly add a small amount of the oil mixture and blend, then add a little more and blend. Do this until the whole mixture is blended. Once both are mixed, continue to blend for a bit, maybe a minute or so, until the mixture looks like white frosting. The mixture, which is now cream, will continue to thicken as it sets.

What if I mess up?
If you mess up and the mixture doesn't emulsify properly, you can do the following:

Pour off the water (you may have to scoop out a teaspoon of oil base to reveal the water).

Put the water in a separate container from the oil.

Warm both up again. When they cool to close to the same temperature, place the water into the blender and slowly add the oil again as you blend.

Or to make it even easier for yourself, you can shake vigorously before using.

Variation 1: Under-Eye Cream
Add 1 teaspoon carrot seed and 1 teaspoon borage oil to the oil group (both

can be found at a health food store). Add the following essential oils to the water group, a drop or two of each: Neroli (Citrus aurantium) EO and Cypress (Cupressus sempervirens) EO. Add no more than five drops for the mixture. Continue to follow the Basic Cream directions.

Variation 2: Foot Cream
Add an additional Tablespoon of mango butter or shea butter to the oil group. Add to the water group 2 drops each of these essential oils: Peppermint (Mentha piperita) and Lavender (Lavandula angustifolia). Make the Foot Cream as you would the Basic Cream.

Variation 3: Body Lotion
How thick you want your lotion is a personal choice; so I am going to give basic suggestions that you can modify as time goes by. The basic variation is as follows: add 2 extra Tablespoons water to the water group and 1 additional Tablespoon of Aloe Vera

As time goes on and as you become more experienced, you can make it with more liquid oils and less hard oils, and more floral waters, teas, and herbal oil infusions. Some great essential oils to add would be Lavender, Rose, Ylang-Ylang (Cananga odorata var genuina), Sandalwood (Santalum album) or Jasmine (Jasminum grandiflorum). You can use cleaned lotion bottles or smaller shampoo bottles. Have a lotion-making party and make the lotion with friends. Give the prepared lotions as gifts. Make nice labels and wrap with raffia and ribbon and you have a finished, very special, and personalized gift. Following these recipes will give you plenty of lotion.

You will also find many infused oil recipes throughout the book also.

Lotion Bars
Lotion Bar is a solid lotion, which you just roll onto the skin.
These are extremely popular!

Easy Lotion Bar
4 oz. beeswax
2 oz. almond oil
2 oz. cocoa butter
1-5 drops Lavender (Lavandula angustifolia), Patchouli (Pogostemon cablin), and Palma Rosa.

Melt the waxes and butters in a double boiler.

When it is completely melted remove from heat and add the almond oil. Then add your essential oils and mix. Pour into containers. Some people like using muffin tins, candy molds, or other kitchen molds or deodorant or large lip balm tubes.

Extra Rich Lotion Bar

6 oz. beeswax

2 oz. mango butter

2 oz. Shea butter

2 oz. almond oil

2 oz. jojoba oil

2 oz. hemp oil or coconut oil

20 drops Essential oil.

In a double boiler add the beeswax shredded, Shea Butter, and the Mango Butter. Allow them to slowly melt, when they are almost all melted add the others oils and mix together. Remove from heat.

Add your essential oil, pour into molds, and allow them to cool and harden.

Emotional Massage Oils
Balancing Oil

Fill a jar with one part of each:

Brahmi (Sida cordifolia)

Guduchi (Tinospora cordifolia)

Shatavari (Asparagus racemosus)

Manjista (Rubia cordifolia)

Half a part of each:

Passionflower (Passiflora incarnata)

Licorice Root (Glycyrrhiza glabra)

Coriander (Coriandrum sativum)

Musta (Cyperus rotundus)

Lavender (Lavandula angustifolia)

Cover the herb in the jar with equal parts of Sesame and Grapeseed oil. Allow this oil to infuse for 2-3 weeks, strain and decant.

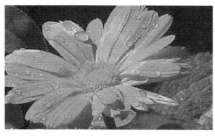

Closeness Oil

This infused oil can help encourage closeness and arousal.

This can also be used as a vaginal lubricant, just not with latex condoms.

In a pint jar fill it with the following oils 3/4 of the jar should contain Sweet Almond oil and the 1/4 should be jojoba oil.

1 part Calendula (Calendula officinalis) flower

1 part Plantain (Plantago major) Leaf

1/2 part Marshmallow (Althaea officinalis) root

20 drops vitamin E oil.

Use in a sensual couples massage.

Citrus Massage Oil

4 oz. Sweet Almond Oil

30 drops Sweet Orange (Citrus sinensis) EO

15 drops Lemon (Citrus limon) EO

10 drops Lime (Citrus aurantifolia) EO

10 drops Grapefruit (Citrus paradisi) EO

10 drops Bergamot (Citrus bergamia) EO

Mix all ingredients together to create a refreshing and energizing oil that is especially kind to dry skin.

Note, please do not apply this oil and go out in the sun afterwards; some citrus EOs including Sweet Orange (Citrus sinensis) can have a phototoxic effect.

Also, people with sensitive skin should try a spot test for this oil first to test for any adverse reactions, this should be done with all applications one makes on their skin.

Sweetest Dreams Massage Oil

4 drops Clary Sage (Salvia sclarea)EO

3 drops Ylang-Ylang (Cananga odorata var genuina)EO

5 drops Neroli (Citrus aurantium) EO

2 drops Patchouli (Pogostemon cablin) EO

Place in 1/4 cup fractionated coconut oil or your favorite carrier oil, or infused oil and then rub slowly and softly.

Cleansing Breath Massage Oil

4 oz. Carrier Oil

10 drops Lavender (Lavendula officinalis) EO
10 Drops Clary Sage (Salvia sclarea) EO
10 drops Eucalyptus (Eucalyptus globulus) EO
3 drops Cajuput EO
Many like this oil for deep breathing. Massage into your chest and upper back area.

Massage Oil- Irritability
In 4 oz. Carrier oil add
10 drops Sandalwood (Santalum album) EO
5 drops Nutmeg (Myristica fragrans) EO
8 drops Petitgrain (Citrus aurantium) EO
Massage into wrists and back of ears when feeling really irritable.

Lack of Energy Massage Oil
2 oz. Carrier Oil EO
10 drops Grapefruit (Citrus paradisi) EO
10 drops Sweet Orange (Citrus sinensis) EO
Massage on the back of neck, knees for a more uplifted feeling.

Erotic Oils
Sweet Sex
½ cup almond oil
10 drops Ylang-Ylang (Cananga odorata var genuina) EO
5 Drops Patchouli (Pogostemon cablin) EO
2 drops Sandalwood (Santalum album) EO
This will warm and inspire. Massage on back, thighs, and the nape of the neck and around the breasts.

Hot Sex
½ cup almond oil (you could also us apricot, grape seed or another carrier oil)
4 drops Black Pepper (Piper nigrum) EO
4 drops Jasmine (Jasminum grandiflorum) EO
4 drops Ylang-Ylang (Cananga odorata var genuina) EO
This is hot!! It makes your skin warm and it lights that fire inside.
Massage into the thighs, use a nice firm massage and pay particular attention to the inner thighs and buttocks.

Exotic Nights

½ cup almond oil (you could also us apricot, grape seed or another carrier oil)

5 drops Sandalwood (Santalum album) EO

5 drops Neroli (Citrus aurantium) EO

3 drops Nutmeg EO

This will inspire the "pirate princess" in you or erotic priestess.

For Him

½ cup almond oil (you could also us apricot, grape seed or another carrier oil)

3 drops Lavender (Lavandula angustifolia)

2 drops Vanilla

5 drops Clary Sage

Causes a semi erotic stupor.

Joyful Sensuality

½ cup almond oil (you could also us apricot, grape seed or another carrier oil)

5 drops Neroli (Citrus aurantium)

3 drops Mandarin

5 drops Vanilla

Use as a massage oil.

3 EVERYTHING BATH

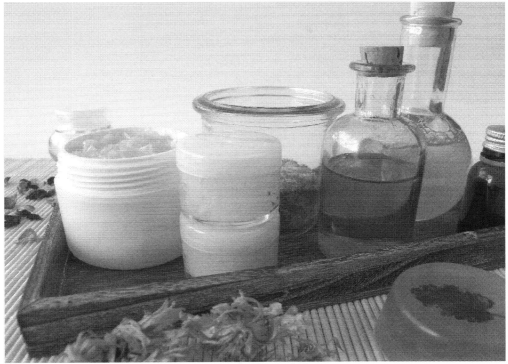

Heiki Rau/Shutterstock

BATH SALTS

The use of salt in healing stretches back to the beginning of time. The earliest systematic description of the different kinds of salts, its uses, and the methods of its extraction was published in China around 2700 years BCE. The healer Hippocrates encouraged his companion healers to offer as a cure for many issues immersion in sea water. The ancient Greeks continued this, and it is still considered healthy to sea bathe. Dr. Charles Russel published "The Uses of Sea Water" in 1753. Many healing modality texts have spoken of the benefits of sea bathing for hundreds of years. Taking the waters, hydrotherapy, are all common types of using baths to heal.

Essentially bath salts are salt, different types of salt and scent. If you want to add a little moisture to your bath you can add a teaspoon oil, like olive, sesame, coconut well mixed in. If you want them to have bubbles, you can add soap flakes, or liquid soap. You can add ground herbs that are powdered, oatmeal and herbal teas to make therapeutic baths.

Many of these sea salt recipes have been part of my recipe collection for years. I have been using and teaching these recipes since 1998.

The following is a list of commonly available salts that are often used when making bath salts. Sea salts and Dead Sea salts are generally available in a variety of grain sizes. Mixing grain sizes can add texture and visual interest to bath salts. Bath salts made with larger salt crystals do look pretty, but they will take longer to dissolve in bathwater. Make sure if using larger crystals that they are completely dissolved before sitting in the bath, so the salt doesn't feel jagged and rough on your bum.

Sea Salts: Sea salts are mineral-rich "all purpose" salts commonly added to bath salt blends. Next to Epsom salts, sea salts are the most inexpensive salts available. They help to draw toxins from the skin and soothe sore muscles. Sea salts are easy to find, most Asian markets sell them in 5 and 10 pound bags, you can also find sea salts in grocery stores and health food stores.

Dead Sea Salts: Dead Sea salts generally have a higher mineral concentration than conventional sea salts. Dead Sea salts can assist in relieving muscular aches and pains, reduce stiffness after exertion, relax muscles and relieve skin complications such as acne, eczema and psoriasis. Dead Sea salts are often coveted by sufferers of skin issues because they sooth these kinds of skin issues so well.

Epsom: Epsom salts are the most affordable and readily available salts, you can get them in most grocery or drug stores. They are often used to help ease muscle tension and joint discomfort. Epsom salts are a fine white crystal powder that can be purchased in any drugstore. They are hydrated magnesium sulfate. Soaking in these salts is soothing to sore muscles because the salts are mildly astringent. They are also used as a laxative (when taken internally) and as an anti-inflammatory soak. Epsom salts are often the go-to salts for athletes, the salts sooth and relax tired and worn out muscles.

Exotic Salts: Other more exotic salts such as Hawaiian Red Sea Salts (Alaea), Black Sea Pink Salts, and Icelandic Geo-Thermal Brine Salts are also available.

These salts generally are more expensive, but their coloration, texture and therapeutic properties are highly sought after. Having bathed in the Red Sea I can attest to the healing power of the salts, they made my skin feel so soft and rejuvenated.

I really feel that I understood the real healing power of sea salt bath after I had my first son. Relaxing and floating in the bath was heavenly. But I was wrong, I truly experienced the power of salt water when I was floating in the Red Sea, I was as peaceful as I had ever been in my life. I am no salt water novice, I have swam in the Pacific Ocean, Atlantic, Caribbean Sea, Red Sea, Mediterranean Sea, Labrador Sea, Gulf of Alaska and the Gulf of Mexico.

You can by looking online find stores that essentially just sell sea salts and types of sea salts. Some are soft, some are crystalline and others are almost a moist powder. You will eventually find the salt that will become your favorite.

In all of these recipes EO means essential oils. In some cases I write it out and in others I just use EO.
All bath salts should be stored in air tight containers and properly labeled. If a reaction occurs, sometimes it can happen, remove your body from the bath and rinse off immediately.

Bath Salts- Basic Base Recipe
2 parts Sea Salt any type, your choice.
2 Parts Borax, Mineral Salts
1 part Epsom Salts
1/4 part powdered herb matter like Lavender (Lavendula officinalis) or Rosemary (Rosmarinus officinalis) (optional)
A few drops essential oil, like Lavender (Lavendula officinalis), Rosemary (Rosmarinus officinalis) or other oils like Rose (Rosa damascene), Sandalwood (Santalum album), Palmarosa (Cymbopogon martini), Rosewood (Aniba rosaeodora) and other oils you like.
EO guideline 15 drops per cup of bath salts. As you learn what you prefer you can modify the Essential oil amount.
Most baths require between a ½ cup to one cups of prepared salts.

Bath Salt Recipes
Soothing Bath Salts
2 pounds Epsom salts
1 pound sea salt

1/2 pound Dead Sea salts
1 1/2 cups vegetable glycerin
1/4 ounce Lavender (Lavendula officinalis) EO
1/16 ounce Helichrysum (Helichrysum angustifolia) EO
1/16 ounce Geranium (Pelargonium graveolens) EO
1/4 ounce baking soda

Mix all dry ingredients together. Place EOs in glycerin and let set for one hour. Add glycerin mixture in salts and knead well. Let set for 24 hours and knead again. Use 1/4 to 1/2 cup per bath.

Energizing Bath Salts

1cup Epsom salts
1cup Mineral Salts (Borax)
1 cup Sea Salt
10-20 drops green food coloring (optional) some people really prefer color therapy also.
6 drops Eucalyptus (Eucalyptus globulus) EO
10 drops Rosemary (Rosmarinus officinalis) EO
15 drops Peppermint (Mentha piperita) EO

Mix salts in large bowl. In smaller bowl take 1/4-1/2 cup salt mixture and add food coloring and oils. Mix WELL. Add back into rest of salt mixture.
Blend all ingredients together well and use a quarter cup in your bath.

Therapeutic Bath Salts

6 cups Epsom salts
2 cups baking soda
1 cup sea salt
40 drops Eucalyptus
30 drops Sweet Orange (Citrus sinensis)
30 drops Lavender (Lavandula angustifolia).

Combine all ingredients in a large jar with lid, shake until thoroughly blended. Make sure you store in an airtight container.

Therapeutic Bath Salts II

These salts are wonderful for sore muscles and overall use, you can add your favorite essential oils.
6 cups Epsom salts
2 cups baking soda

1 cup sea salt
Combine all ingredients in a large jar with lid, shake until thoroughly blended. Store salts into a decorative container and use ½- 1 cup at a time. This is the unscented blend I make for my two sons. Both are huge, muscular defensive linemen who play football, and they can take a hit, but sometimes a soak is really needed, and this is my go-to blend. Many of their football buddies also like this recipe.

Muscle Relaxing Bath
2 cups sea salt
1 cup mineral salts
5 drops Black Pepper (Piper nigrum) Essential Oil
5 drops Cypress (Cupressus sempervirens) Essential Oil
Combine in an airtight container and use as need. ½ cup at a time.

Sinus Headache Bath Salts
2-3 cups Epsom salts
1 cup Mineral Salts
1/3 cup Peppermint (Mentha piperita) leaf, powdered
1/3 cup Spearmint (Mentha spicata) leaf, powdered
10 drops Peppermint (Mentha piperita) EO
20 drops Rosemary (Rosmarinus officinalis) EO
10 drops Eucalyptus (Eucalyptus globulus) EO
Blend well and use a ¼ cup in your bath.

Oatmeal Bath Salts
1 cup borax
1/8 cup kelp powder
1/8 cup finely ground oatmeal
1/8 cup sea salt
Place all in a glass jar. To this add your favorite finely powdered aromatic herbs to the salt mixture and mix well or add several drops of your favorite essential oil/oils. Let sit for several hours or overnight to dry and allow oils to penetrate salts. Break up any lumps that formed when adding the oil. Store in an airtight container. Add about ¼ cup to bathwater as desired.

Oatmeal Therapeutic Bath Salts 1 cup Epsom salts
1/8 cup powdered Plantain (Plantago major) leaf

1/8 cup finely ground oatmeal

1/8 cup sea salt

1 tsp. green clay

Place all ingredients a glass jar. To this add your favorite finely powdered aromatic herbs to the salt mixture and mix well or add several drops of your favorite essential oil/oils. Let sit for at least several hours or overnight to dry and allow oils to penetrate salts. Break up any lumps that formed when adding the oil. Store in an airtight container. Add about 4 Tbsp. to bathwater as desired.

Menstruation Sea Salt Bath

These salts are wonderful for PMS and menstrual issues, like tension, headaches, and retaining water.

2 cups Sea Salt

1 Cup Epsom Salts

1 tablespoon Green Clay

10 drops Roman Chamomile (Matricaria chamomilla)

2 drops Fennel (Foeniculum vulgare) Essential Oil

Combine in an airtight container and use as need. ½ cup at a time.

Milk Baths
Milk Bath Salts

7 oz. Epsom salts

2 oz. powdered milk

2 oz. Borax (Mineral Salts)

2 oz. Sodium Bicarbonate

2 oz. Sea Salt (medium NOT coarse)

2 oz. Irish Sea Salt

1 1/2 teaspoon Vegetable Glycerin

1/2 teaspoon Essential oil- use

Mix all of the salts together and then drizzle over the glycerin and essential oil. Combine well.

Lavender, Lemon (Citrus limon): 12 drops Lavender (Lavandula angustifolia) essential oil, 9 drops Lemon (Citrus limon), and 2 drops chamomile

Uplifting 10 drops Bergamot (Citrus bergamia) EO, 9 drops Grapefruit (Citrus paradisi) EO, 2 drops Palmarosa, 2 drops Ylang-Ylang (Cananga odorata var genuina).

Use in the evening, or when you can limit sun exposure. The citrus can increase the likely hood of sunburn.

Spicy 10 drops Mandarin EO, 10 drops Patchouli (Pogostemon cablin), 1 drop Clove EO

Some people are sensitive to clove, if that is the case you can leave it out, and add a drop of Sandalwood (Santalum album) instead.

Roses are Red- 10 drops Rose absolute, 2 drops Palmarosa

Oatmeal Milk Bath

2 cups Epsom salts

1 cup Sea salt

1/2 cup nonfat powdered milk

1/2 cup oatmeal ground to a very fine powder in a food processor.

15 drops Patchouli (Pogostemon cablin) EO

15 drops Clary Sage (Salvia sclarea) EO

15 drops Cedarwood (Cedrus atlantica) EO

Use 1/3 cup per bath.

Sweet Emotions Milk Bath

1/2 cup Celtic Sea Salt

1 cup Powdered Milk

1 cup Epsom Salts

1 cup Sea Salt

1 cup Mineral Salts

10 drops Ylang Ylang (Cananga odorata) EO

5 drops Bergamot (Citrus bergamia) EO

10 drops Lavender (Lavendula officinalis) EO

5 drops Peppermint (Mentha piperita) EO

5 drops Ginger (Zingiber officinale) EO

10 drops Cedarwood (Cedrus atlantica) EO

10 drops Tangerine (Citrus reticulata) EO

10 drops Orange (Citrus sinensis) EO

Add a ¼ cup-a 1/3 cup to your bath. Make sure because the salts are so rich in essential oils the salts need to be well mixed in.

Fragrant Bath Salts

1 cup instant nonfat dry milk

1 cup baking soda

2 Tablespoon cornstarch

1 cup sea salt
1 Tablespoon cream of tartar
1 Tablespoon cinnamon powder
2 vanilla beans
Combine all and store in a decorative container in the bathroom. Add as much as desired to your bath water. Leave the vanilla beans in the jar.

Insomnia Milk Bath
1 Tablespoon. Almond oil
4 drops Lavender (Lavendula officinalis) EO
3 drops Marjoram (Origanum majorana) EO
2 drops Benzoin (Styrax tonkinesis) EO
1 cup of powdered milk
Pour oils into a small bowl, mix thoroughly. Stir in 1 cup of powdered milk. Add mixture to bath water.

Insomnia Milk Bath II
4 tbsp. Grapeseed oil
10 drops Lavender (Lavandula angustifolia) EO
6 drops Marjoram EO
5 drops Chamomile essential oil
1 cup of powdered milk
1 cup sea salt
Pour oils into a small bowl, mix thoroughly. Stir in 1 cup of powdered milk. Add mixture to hot bath water, swoosh around to disperse the oils and ingredients.

Honey Dreams Bath
1 cup honey
1 cup boiling water
2 cups milk
1/2 cup sea salt
2 Tbsp. baking soda
10 drops Lavender (Lavandula angustifolia)
10 drops Cedarwood (Cedrus atlantica)
Dissolve sea salt and baking soda in bathwater. Dissolve honey in boiling water, add milk. Add milk and honey mixture to bathwater. Add vanilla.

Milk and Honey Bath

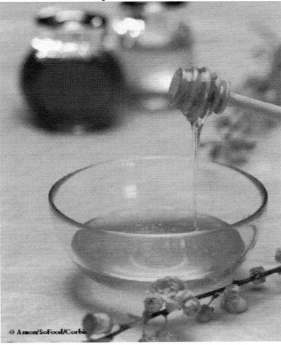

1 cup honey
1 cup boiling water
2 cups milk
1/2 cup sea salt
2 Tablespoons baking soda
10 drops of vanilla oil
Dissolve sea salt and baking soda in bathwater. Dissolve honey in boiling water, add milk. Add milk, vanilla and honey mixture to bathwater. Swish the water around and enjoy. Many people with skin issues really like this bath. The honey can feel really healing to the skin.

Salt Scrubs
Lavender Salt Scrub
1 cup Pink Himalayan sea salt, or finer Celtic sea salt.
½ cup oil like Almond, Apricot or Olive Oil.
10-15 drops Lavender (Lavandula angustifolia) essential oil
Rub into damp skin or spread on loofah or washcloth, and use as all over body scrub when needed. Salt scrubs are usually too harsh for the fragile skin on our faces.

Energizing Sea Salt Scrub
1 cup Pink Himalayan sea salt, or finer Celtic sea salt.
½ cup oil like Almond, Apricot or Olive Oil.
10 drops peppermint essential oil
Rub into damp skin or spread on loofah or washcloth, and use as all over body scrub when needed.

Gentle Life Sea Salt Scrub
1 cup Pink Himalayan sea salt, or finer Celtic sea salt.

½ cup ground oatmeal
½ cup oil like Almond, Apricot or Olive Oil.
Rub into damp skin or spread on loofah or washcloth, and use as all over body scrub when needed.

Oatmeal and Almond Body Scrub

1/4 cup finely ground oatmeal
1/4 cup finely ground almonds
1 teaspoon Myrrh (Commiphora myrrha) Powder
2 tablespoons Witch Hazel
1 teaspoon Glycerin
2 tablespoons fine sea salt
Mix well. Store in refrigerator. Mix well, and use as you would as traditional scrub.

Soapy Salt Scrub

1/2 cup Sea Salt
1/2 cup Sweet Almond oil
1/2 oz. plain melted glycerin soap or liquid castile soap
Mix first two ingredients
Melt soap
Whisk into salt, almond oil
2 drops Tea Tree (Melaleuca alternifolia) EO
2 drops Lavender (Lavandula angustifolia) EO
Mix well, and use as you would as traditional scrub.

Peppermint Foot Scrub

Combine all in a bowl and mix well.
1 cup Epsom salt
1 cup Sea salt (your choice of variety)
1 cup Baking Soda (1 cup)
2 tablespoons Olive Oil
20 drops Peppermint Essential Oil
20 drops Tea Tree (Melaleuca alternifolia) Essential Oil
Pour all ingredients into glass jar and shake to mix. Use weekly to scrub feet and soothe rough heels. This often works best after soaking in a hot bath for 20 minutes of soaking your feet to soften rough, thick skin.

Sea Salt Body Polisher

1 cup extra-fine sea salt- you can run this in the blender to make it extra fine.
1/2 cup Jojoba oil
¼ cup Rose hip oil
1/2-cup liquid soap
10 drops Neroli (Citrus aurantium)
Mix well together and use as a body polish. Apply to skin and then rinse off.

Bath Oils

Generally bath oils all you need per bath is 1 teaspoon to 1 tablespoon of oil. A little oil goes a really long way. Make sure you mix the oil into the bath water, to disperse the oil.

Enlightened Bath Oil

1/4 cup Carrier oil
20 drops Sandalwood (Santalum album)
10 drops Jasmine (Jasminum grandiflorum) EO
10 drops Rose EO
5 drops Bergamot (Citrus bergamia) EO
Add a teaspoon or two to the bath.

Sensual Bath Oil

1/2 cup of base Carrier oil
20 drops Jasmine (Jasminum grandiflorum) EO
10 drops Sweet Orange (Citrus sinensis) EO
10 drops Rose EO
Add a teaspoon or two to the bath.

Revitalizing Oil

1/2 cup Carrier oil
20 drops Geranium (Pelargonium graveolens) EO
10 drops Lemon (Citrus limon) EO
10 drops Clary Sage (Salvia sclarea) EO
Add a teaspoon or two to the bath.

Relaxing Oil

1/2 cup carrier oil
12 drops Sandalwood (Santalum album) EO

10 drops Orange EO
15 drops Clary Sage (Salvia sclarea) EO
Add a teaspoon or two to the bath.

Lavender Alcohol Based Bath Oil

1/2 cup Carrier Oil
1/8 cup vodka
20 drops Lavender (Lavandula angustifolia) EO
Pour in a glass bottle and allow it to mature for two weeks, gently shaking to mix every day.
Add 2 tablespoons to the bath and mix in to full tub.

Rose Alcohol Based Bath Oil

1/2 cup Carrier Oil
1/8 cup vodka
10 drops Rose Absolute
10 drops Palmarosa EO
Pour in a glass bottle and allow it to mature for two weeks, gently shaking to mix every day.
Add 2 tablespoons to the bath and mix in to full tub.

Relaxing Alcohol Based Bath Oil

1/2 cup Carrier Oil
1/8 cup vodka
10 drops Clary Sage (Salvia sclarea) EO
10 drops Lavender (Lavandula angustifolia) EO
Pour in a glass bottle and allow it to mature for two weeks, gently shaking to mix every day.
Add 2 tablespoons to the bath and mix in to full tub.

Sore Muscle Alcohol Based Bath Oil

1/2 cup Carrier Oil
1/8 cup vodka
10 drops Peppermint EO
10 drops Rosemary (Rosmarinus officinalis) EO
10 drops Eucalyptus EO
Pour in a glass bottle and allow it to mature for two weeks, gently shaking to mix every day.

Add 2 tablespoons to the bath and mix in to full tub.

Sleepytime Bath Oil Blend
5 drops Bergamot (Citrus bergamia) EO
4 drops Lemon (Citrus limon) EO
4 drops Pine (Pinus sylvestris) EO
2 drop Cedarwood (Cedrus atlantica) EO
5 drop Mandarin EO
½ cup Grapeseed, Borage seed or other light oil.
Mix the essential oils into the

DeStress and Rest Bath Oil
20 drops Lavender (Lavandula angustifolia) EO
10 drops Cedarwood (Cedrus atlantica) EO
30 drops Tangerine EO
10 drops Clary Sage (Salvia sclarea)
1 cup of jojoba, hazelnut, sunflower, or Grapeseed oil
Mix well and use 1-2 tablespoons per bath. Or further dilute with at least another ½ cup of oil and use as a massage oil.

Vanilla Bath Oil
1 cup Grapeseed oil
1/2 cup castile soap
1 Tbsp. real vanilla extract
1 split vanilla bean
1/4 cup honey
Blend all ingredients together, except the vanilla bean. Add the vanilla bean. Allow the salts to sit for 2 weeks before using. Shake well before using. Use 1/4 cup per bath.

Single Bath Oils
Here are some essential oils that can be added singularly to the bath. These oils are helpful for the following issues. Add to a full bath, swish well and incorporate into the water before getting in, if the bath is not full then reduce the amount of drops added.

Bergamot (Citrus bergamia) EO for depression, our cloudy outlook – 7 drops

Chamomile EO for insomnia, feeling cranky, itchy or irritated skin – 9 drops

Clary Sage (Salvia sclarea) EO- Intense relaxation, releasing stress and tension. 7-10 drops.

Frankincense EO for sedative feelings, relieving anxiety, calming and relaxing, relieving stress – 8 drops

Grapefruit (Citrus paradisi) EO for burnout and stress, anxiousness, - 5 drops

Jasmine (Jasminum grandiflorum) EO for lethargy, stress, fatigue and feeling stuck, also works to promote sensual feelings. – 8-10 drops

Lavender (Lavandula angustifolia) EO positive, soothing and relaxing, combat insomnia – 10 drops

Palmarosa EO for relaxing yet uplifting and energizing – 12 drops
Patchouli (Pogostemon cablin) for energizing and stimulating – 7-10 drops

Rose Absolute-for happiness and pleasure, promotes well-being, an a sense of romance and love – 10 drops

Rosewood EO Mood supporting, relaxing, calming and supporting, soothes feelings of being overwhelmed and easing the spirit. - 5-7 drops

Sandalwood (Santalum album) EO for sensual feelings, warm love, aphrodisiac feeling, feelings of comfort and safety. – 8- 10 drops

Ylang Ylang (Cananga odorata) EO helpful for anxiety, depressive feelings and stress- 10 drops

Bubble Bath
You can use a bubble bath base, or castile soap for any of these recipes. Use 1-2 tablespoons per bath. You may want to add a few additional drops of EO to the mixture, but try it first with the listed amounts. You don't want to make it to strong.

Moisturizing Bubble Bath
1 cup Castile soap or bubble bath base
10 drops vitamin E
10 drops Olive Oil, Grapeseed oil, almond oil
Mix the essential oils into the soap. Use 2-3 tablespoons per bath

Lavender Moisturizing Bubble Bath
1 cup Castile soap or bubble bath base
10 drops Vitamin E
10 drops Olive Oil
10 drops Lavender (Lavandula angustifolia) EO
Mix the essential oils into the soap. Use 2-3 tablespoons per bath

Sunshine Bubble Bath
1 cup Castile soap or bubble bath base
10 drops Vitamin E
10 drops Grapefruit EO
10 drops Peppermint (Mentha piperita) EO
2 drops Black Pepper (Piper nigrum) EO
Mix the essential oils into the soap. Use 2-3 tablespoons per bath.

Sore Muscle Bubble Bath
1 cup Castile soap or bubble bath base
10 drops vitamin E
20 drops Rosemary (Rosmarinus officinalis) EO
10 drops Pine (Pinus sylvestris) EO
10 drops Peppermint (Mentha piperita) EO
Mix well, add 2-3 tablespoons your bath and soak away sore muscles. For extra relief add a cup of Epsom salts to the bath.

Bath Teas
Bath teas are teas that are made in large pots allowed to cool and added to the bath. Generally a bath tea is made in a stock pot. I like to add the whole pot of tea, strained to my baths. The amount of herb used is individual. Many people just use a tablespoon or two of each for ease. I generally like to use total one cup of herbs per gallon of water. Add the herbs to the water, bring to a boil and allow to cool and strain.

Calming Tea Bath
Equal parts of, for instance for enough for one bath use
Chamomile Flowers
Lavender Flowers
Rose Petals
Blend all together and make as a tea. 1 cup per two gallons of water. Strain and add to the bath. You can also add orange peel or Lemon Balm (Melissa officinalis) also.

Stimulating Tea Bath
Equal parts of
Peppermint Leaves
Eucalyptus Leaves
Lavender Flowers
Blend all together and make as a tea. 1 cup per two gallons of water. Strain and add to the bath. You can also use Rosemary, or Birch leaves also.

Floral Tea Bath
Equal Parts of
Jasmine Flowers
Rose Petals
Orange Peels
Blend all together and make as a tea. 1 cup per two gallons of water. Strain and add to the bath. You can also use bee balm flower, orange blossom, or chrysanthemums.

Muscle Soothing Tea
Peppermint Leaf
Pine
Lavender Flower
Blend all together and make as a tea. 1 cup per two gallons of water. Strain and add to the bath. You can also use Spearmint (Mentha spicata), Black Pepper (Piper nigrum), Cedar fronds or Bee Balm.

Stress Relief Tea
Spearmint Leaf
Rosemary

Lavender Flower
Sage
Blend all together and make as a tea. 1 cup per two gallons of water. Strain and add to the bath.

Stress Relief Tea II
Lemon Verbena
Lavender Flowers
Calendula (Calendula officinalis) Petals
Lemon Balm
Blend all together and make as a tea. 1 cup per two gallons of water. Strain and add to the bath.

Mud Baths
When making a mud bath you can do one of two options.
1. Make the mud bath, mix with water to thin, and make a paste, cover body and allow it to dry for 10 minutes and then take a shower or bath to remove the mud.
2. Mix the mud bath, and add it to a full bathtub, and take a bath. When finished rinse off in the shower to remove the mud mixture.

Cleansing and Detox Mud Bath
1 cup green clay powder
10 drops Chamomile EO
Add the clay and EO to a full bath, mix in the clay. It will turn your water green with the clay, it feels really nice though as it cleans out your pores. Rinse off in the shower after you are done the bath.

Pink Mud Bath
1 cup pink clay powder
¼ cup powdered Rose petals.
¼ cup rosewater
Add the clay and rosewater to a full bath, mix in the clay. It will turn your water green with the clay, it feels really nice though as it cleans out your pores. Rinse off in the shower after you are done the bath.

Acne Blend Mud Paint

1 cup Pink, White or Green Clay
¼ cup Witch Hazel
¼ teaspoon Rose Hydrosol EO
20 drops Tea Tree EO
20 drops Lavender EO

Make into a paste adding water until you have the consistency you need. Paint over back acne with the back of a spoon. Allow to dry and rinse off in a bath.

Misc. Baths
Mint Bath

1 cup fresh Spearmint (Mentha spicata) simmered
½ cup Oatmeal
5 drops Peppermint (Mentha piperita) Essential oil

Simmer the finely ground oatmeal and fresh Spearmint for 15 minutes in 5 cups of water.

Strain, add the essential oil and pour into bath. Make sure the prepared bath is finely dispersed into the bath water...

Athlete's Foot Sea Salt Soak

In a foot bath filled with hot water place ¼ cup sea salt
20 drops Tea Tree (Melaleuca alternifolia) EO
5 drops Myrrh (Commiphora myrrha) Tincture

Soak the feet 2-3 times a day for 3-5 days, and then once a day for a week.

4 BODY SPRAYS

Body mists can be therapeutic, or used just as a fragrance for the body. Everyone has their own sense of smell and what they like in a fragrance. Feel free to alter and make the scent one you like.

All of the body mists listed here are all made to be dispersed in water. If you want you can add a teaspoon vodka for preservation. When using a body spray mist your skin, avoiding the face and genitals. If using as a room mist, you just gently spray a few mists into the air. If you are making a body oil you can add the essential oils to a carrier oil instead of water. Use the same amount of oil, as you would water. So if the recipe requires 2 oz. water, replace it with 2 oz. of carrier oil.

Energy Booster
14 drops Orange (Citrus sinensis) EO
10 drops Rosemary (Rosmarinus officinalis) EO
10 drops Grapefruit (Citrus paradisi) EO
Add to a 4 oz. Mister, or use as a diffusion blend, without the water.
Add the essential oils to the mister bottle and then add the water, cap and shake well. Mist body, or area around you.

Relaxation and Rest
15 drops Lavender (Lavendula officinalis) EO
10 drops Roman Chamomile (Matricaria chamomilla) EO
15 drops Clary Sage (Salvia sclarea) EO
Add to a 4 oz. Mister, or use as a diffusion blend, without the water.
Add the essential oils to the mister bottle and then add the water, cap and shake well. Mist your body, or the area around you. I like this blend for when I come home from a long birth and I need to relax.

Uplifting/Postpartum Blend
20 drops Orange (Citrus sinensis) EO
15 drops Grapefruit (Citrus paradisi) EO
10 drops Ylang Ylang (Cananga odorata) EO
Add to a 4 oz. Mister, or use as a diffusion blend, without the water.
Add the essential oils to the mister bottle and then add the water, cap and shake well. This blend is wonderful for when you are feeling tired or needing a lift during the postpartum period.

Enhancing Self-Love
10 drops Rose otto EO
10 drops Jasmine (Jasminum grandiflorum) otto EO
Add to a 4 oz. Mister, or use as a diffusion blend, without the water.
Add the essential oils to the mister bottle and then add the water, cap and shake well.

Coping with New Responsibilities- Great for the overwhelmed Mom or Dad.
20 drops Rosemary (Rosmarinus officinalis) EO
10 drops Cypress (Cupressus sempervirens) EO
10 drops Cedarwood (Cedrus atlantica) EO
Add to a 4 oz. Mister, or use as a diffusion blend, without the water.
Add the essential oils to the mister bottle and then add the water, cap and shake well.

Sinus Mist
This is helpful with a sinus infection or clogged, sore sinuses.
4 oz. Water
25 drops Rosemary (Rosmarinus officinalis) EO
15 drops Thyme (Thymus vulgaris) EO
10 drops Ravensara (Ravensara aromatica) EO
Mist around house and face. Not directly at the face.
Add to a 4 oz. Mister, or use as a diffusion blend, without the water.
Add the essential oils to the mister bottle and then add the water, cap and shake well.

Essential Oil Blends for Emotional Issues
How to Use These Blends
Mist
Make a room mist, for the environment or for the air in general, as a deodorizer or a therapeutic addition to a room. You can also use these blends in a 2-4 oz. mister bottle, as a body mist or a room mist.

Massage oil
For a massage oil add the essential oil to 2-4 ounces of a carrier oil, like almond or apricot kernel oil.
When making the blend start out with 2 oz. and if you need to dilute the blend, add more water or carrier oil.

These blends are synergies and very potent. If you feel a blend is too strong for yourself or a client simply add a more carrier oil, or water.

Absent-mindedness
15 drops Cedarwood (Cedrus atlantica) EO
5 drops Tangerine (Citrus reticulata) EO
1 drop Rosemary (Rosmarinus officinalis) EO

Ageing, feelings of
15 drops Tangerine (Citrus reticulata) EO
5 drops Patchouli (Pogostemon cablin) EO
1 teaspoon Rose Hydrosol

Anger
5 drops Chamomile (Matricaria chamomilla) EO
5 drops Spearmint (Mentha spicata) EO
10 drops Ylang-Ylang (Cananga odorata var genuina) EO

Anxiety
5 drops Cedarwood (Cedrus atlantica) EO
5 drops Clary Sage (Salvia sclarea) EO
5 drops Tangerine (Citrus reticulata) EO
Or
5 drops Sandalwood (Santalum album) EO
5 drops Frankincense (Boswellia carterii) EO

3 drop Lavender (Lavendula officinalis) EO
2 drops Marjoram (Marjorana hortensis) EO

Anxiety, sexual
10 drops Sandalwood (Santalum album) EO
10 drops Ylang-Ylang (Cananga odorata var genuina) EO
2 drops Tangerine (Citrus reticulata) or Sweet Orange (Citrus sinensis) EO

Apathy
4 drops Lemon (Citrus limon) EO
4 drops Orange (Citrus sinensis) EO
2 drops Tea Tree (Melaleuca alternifolia) EO

Bitterness
15 drops Lemon (Citrus limon) EO
4 drops Tangerine (Citrus reticulata) EO

Boredom
10 drops Orange (Citrus sinensis) EO
10 drops Frankincense (Boswellia carterii) EO

Burn-out
15 drops Frankincense (Boswellia carterii) EO
4 drops Sandalwood (Santalum album) EO

Change, coping with
15 drops Ylang-Ylang (Cananga odorata var genuina) EO

Change, difficulty in adjusting to
10 drops Clary Sage (Salvia sclarea) EO
5 drops Lavender (Lavendula officinalis) EO

Change, difficulty in making
10 drops Orange (Citrus sinensis) EO

Claustrophobia
5 drops Clary Sage (Salvia sclarea) EO
5 drops Frankincense (Boswellia carterii) EO

5 drops Bergamot (Citrus bergamia) EO
5 drops Mandarin (Citrus reticulata) EO

Compulsiveness
10 drops Clary Sage (Salvia sclarea) EO
6 drops Frankincense (Boswellia carterii) EO
5 drops Tangerine (Citrus reticulata) EO

Concentration, lack of
10 drops Cedarwood (Cedrus atlantica) EO
5 drops Eucalyptus (Eucalyptus globulus) EO
3 drops Rosemary (Rosmarinus officinalis) EO
Or
8 drops Ylang Ylang (Cananga odorata) EO
8 drops Lemon (Citrus limon) EO
4 drops Basil (Ocimum basilicum) EO

Confidence, lack of
15 drops Ylang-Ylang (Cananga odorata var genuina) EO

Confusion
10 drops Geranium (Pelargonium graveolens) EO
10 drops Lemon (Citrus limon) EO
5 drops Rosemary (Rosmarinus officinalis) EO

Courage, lack of (See also Fear)
15 drops Frankincense (Boswellia carterii) EO

Critical of others
15 drops Rosewood (Aniba rosaeodora) EO

Cynicism
20 drops Sandalwood (Santalum album) EO

Daydreaming
10 drops Cedarwood (Cedrus atlantica) EO
10 drops Rosewood (Aniba rosaeodora) EO

Depression
5 drops Bergamot (Citrus bergamia) EO
5 drops Tangerine (Citrus reticulata) EO
5 drops Orange (Citrus sinensis) EO
Or
5 drops Clary Sage (Salvia sclarea) EO
5 drops Melissa (Melissa officinalis) EO
5 drops Chamomile (Matricaria chamomilla) EO
Or
5 drops Sandalwood (Santalum album) EO
5 drops Lavender (Lavendula officinalis) EO
5 drops Ylang Ylang (Cananga odorata) EO

Despondency
10 drops Juniper (Juniperus communis) EO
5 drops Marjoram EO
5 drops Jasmine (Jasminum grandiflorum) EO
Or
10 drops Cypress (Cupressus sempervirens) EO
5 drops Melissa (Melissa officinalis) EO
5 drops Neroli (Citrus aurantium) EO

Detail, over-preoccupation with
10 drops Juniper (Juniperus communis) EO
5 drops Tea Tree (Melaleuca alternifolia) EO
2 drops Bergamot (Citrus bergamia) EO

Discipline, lack of
10 drops Frankincense (Boswellia carterii) EO
5 drops Ylang Ylang (Cananga odorata) EO

Disorientation
10 drops Rosemary (Rosmarinus officinalis) EO
10 drops Lavender (Lavendula officinalis) EO
5 drops Grapefruit (Citrus paradisi) EO

Dreams, recurrent
10 drops Clary Sage (Salvia sclarea) EO

12 drops Sandalwood (Santalum album) EO

Empathy, lack of
20 drops Rosewood (Aniba rosaeodora)

Emptiness, emotional
20 drops Tangerine (Citrus reticulata) EO

Exhaustion, mental
12 drops Frankincense (Boswellia carterii) EO

Exhaustion, from overwork
10 drops Clary Sage (Salvia sclarea) EO
20 drops Orange (Citrus sinensis) EO

Fatigue, mental
These blends are helpful for parents. Moms and Dads are often so mentally exhausted, they need a little help sometimes.
10 drops Frankincense (Boswellia carterii) EO
10 drops Lavender (Lavendula officinalis) EO
5 drops Spearmint (Mentha spicata) EO
5 drops Rosemary (Rosmarinus officinalis) EO
5 drops Rosewood (Aniba rosaeodora) EO

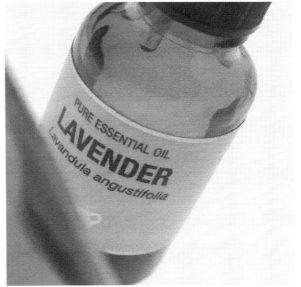

Fear Overall
10 drops Chamomile (Matricaria chamomilla) (both) EO
10 drops Frankincense (Boswellia carterii) EO

Fear, acute
15-20 drops Geranium (Pelargonium graveolens) EO
5 drops Ylang Ylang (Cananga odorata) EO

Fear, of coming events
15 drops Sandalwood (Santalum album) EO
10 drops of Palmarosa (Cymbopogon martini) EO
5 drops Juniper (Juniperus communis) EO

Fear, of confronting issues
3 drops Marjoram EO
3 drops Cedarwood (Cedrus atlantica) EO
3 drops Laurel EO
Or
10 drops Grapefruit (Citrus paradisi) EO
10 drops Rosemary (Rosmarinus officinalis) EO

Fear, of the dark
15 drops Lavender (Lavendula officinalis) EO
5 drops Coriander EO

Fear, of dying
15 drops Tangerine (Citrus reticulata) EO
5 drops Melissa (Melissa officinalis) EO
5 drops Ginger (Zingiber officinale) EO

Fear, of effort
10 drops Sandalwood (Santalum album) EO
15 drops Cedarwood (Cedrus atlantica) EO

Fear, of failure
10 drops Lavender (Lavendula officinalis) EO
5 drops Sandalwood (Santalum album) EO
10 drops Ylang-Ylang (Cananga odorata var genuina) EO

Fear, of going mad
5 drops Ylang-Ylang (Cananga odorata var genuina) EO
5 drops Chamomile (Matricaria chamomilla) EO
5 drops Neroli (Citrus aurantium) EO

Fear, of letting go

15 drops Ylang-Ylang (Cananga odorata var genuina) EO
5 drops Neroli (Citrus aurantium) EO
2 drops Grapefruit (Citrus paradisi) EO

Fear, of people

10 drops Lavender (Lavendula officinalis) EO
10 drops Ylang-Ylang (Cananga odorata var genuina) EO

Fear, of others opinions

10 drops Cypress (Cupressus sempervirens) EO
10 drops Jasmine (Jasminum grandiflorum) EO
5 drops Helichrysum (Helichrysum angustifolia) EO

Fear, rigid with

15 drops Geranium (Pelargonium graveolens) EO
10 drops Rose EO

Fear, of showing feelings

15 drops Marjoram EO
10 drops Ylang-Ylang (Cananga odorata var genuina) EO

Fear, with inner trembling

10 drops Lavender (Lavendula officinalis) EO
5 drops Clary Sage (Salvia sclarea) EO
5 drops Orange (Citrus sinensis) EO

Fear, of unknown origin

5 drops Lavender (Lavendula officinalis) EO
5 drops Clary Sage (Salvia sclarea) EO
5 drops Grapefruit (Citrus paradisi) EO
5 drops Laurel

Frustration

10 drops Ylang-Ylang (Cananga odorata var genuina) EO
5 drops Bergamot (Citrus bergamia) EO
10 drops Lavender (Lavendula officinalis) EO

Giving in to others
10 drops Cypress (Cupressus sempervirens) EO
10 drops Palmarosa (Cymbopogon martini) EO

Grief
10 drops Marjoram (Origanum majorana) EO
10 drops Orange (Citrus sinensis) EO
10 drops Clary Sage (Salvia sclarea) EO

Grief, for long past
10 drops Tangerine (Citrus reticulate) EO
15 drops Grapefruit (Citrus paradisi) EO
5 drops Ravensara (Ravensara aromatica) EO

Grief, prolonged after loss
20 drops Frankincense (Boswellia carterii) EO

Grudge Holding One
15 drops Lemon (Citrus limon) EO
5 drops Melissa (Melissa officinalis) EO
10 drops Grapefruit (Citrus paradisi) EO

Grumpiness
10 drops Redwood EO
5 drops Palmarosa (Cymbopogon martini) EO

Guilt feelings
5 drops Juniper (Juniperus communis) EO
5 drops Ylang-Ylang (Cananga odorata var genuina) EO
10 drops Cardamom (Elettaria cardamomum) EO

Hopelessness
5 drops Orange (Citrus sinensis) EO
10 drops Tangerine (Citrus reticulata) EO
10 drops Mandarin (Citrus reticulata) EO

Hostility
10 drops Clary Sage (Salvia sclarea) EO

10 drops Marjoram (Origanum majorana) EO

Hyperactivity
15 drops Clary- Sage (Salvia sclarea)
5 drops Lavender (Lavendula officinalis)
10 drops Melissa (Melissa officinalis)

Hypersensitivity
2 drops Peppermint (Mentha piperita) EO
5 drops Spearmint (Mentha spicata) EO

Hysteria
10 drops Chamomile (Matricaria chamomilla) EO
10 drops Lavender (Lavendula officinalis) EO
5 Peppermint (Mentha piperita) EO
Or
10 drops Marjoram (Origanum majorana) EO
10 drops Chamomile (Matricaria chamomilla) EO
10 drops Melissa (Melissa officinalis) EO

Impatience
5 drops Chamomile (Matricaria chamomilla) EO
10 drops Lavender (Lavendula officinalis) EO
10 drops Ylang-Ylang (Cananga odorata var genuina) EO

Impulsiveness
15 drops Chamomile (Matricaria chamomilla) EO
5 drops Clary Sage (Salvia sclarea) EO

Indecision
10 drops Rosemary (Rosmarinus officinalis) EO
10 drops Marjoram (Origanum majorana) EO
10 drops Grapefruit (Citrus paradisi) EO

Insecurity
10 drops Juniper (Juniperus communis) EO
5 drops Sandalwood (Santalum album) EO
10 drops Bergamot (Citrus bergamia) EO

Or
5 drops Geranium (Pelargonium graveolens) EO
5 drops Patchouli (Pogostemon cablin) EO
5 drops Jasmine (Jasminum grandiflorum) EO
5 drops Vetiver (Vetiveria zizanoides) EO

Insomnia
10 drops Chamomile (Matricaria chamomilla) EO
5 drops Clary Sage (Salvia sclarea) EO
10 drops Lavender (Lavendula officinalis) EO
15 drops Orange (Citrus sinensis) EO
5 drops Sandalwood (Santalum album) EO
10 drops Tangerine (Citrus reticulata) EO
3 drops Ylang-Ylang (Cananga odorata var genuina) EO

Instability
15 drops Geranium (Pelargonium graveolens) EO
15 drops Rosewood (Aniba rosaeodora) EO

Irrationality
10 drops Lavender (Lavendula officinalis) EO
15 drops Ylang-Ylang (Cananga odorata var genuina) EO

Irritability
5 drops Chamomile (Matricaria chamomilla) EO
5 drops Cypress (Cupressus sempervirens) EO
5 drops Lavender (Lavendula officinalis) EO
5 drops Sandalwood (Santalum album) EO

Jealousy
10 drops Cypress (Cupressus sempervirens) EO
10 drops Ylang-Ylang (Cananga odorata var genuina) EO
5 drops Lemon (Citrus limon) EO
Or
10 drops Helichrysum (Helichrysum angustifolia) EO
10 drops Cedarwood (Cedrus atlantica) EO
10 drops Palmarosa (Cymbopogon martini) EO

Joy, lack of
10 drops Orange (Citrus sinensis) or Mandarin (Citrus reticulata) EO
10 drops Tangerine (Citrus reticulata) EO
10 drops Grapefruit (Citrus paradisi) EO

Lethargy, listlessness
You can use any with a total of twenty five drops for the blend in the 2 tablespoons carrier oil.
10 drops Clary Sage (Salvia sclarea) EO
10 drops Cypress (Cupressus sempervirens) EO
5 drops Juniper (Juniperus communis) EO
Or
10 drops Lemon (Citrus limon) EO
10 drops Orange (Citrus sinensis) EO
2 drops Rosemary (Rosmarinus officinalis) EO
3 drops Sandalwood (Santalum album) EO

Loneliness
You can use any with a total of twenty five drops for the blend in the 2 tablespoons carrier oil.
10 drops Marjoram (Origanum majorana) EO
5 drops Juniper (Juniperus communis) EO
10 drops Clary Sage (Salvia sclarea) EO
Or
10 drops Rosemary (Rosmarinus officinalis) EO
5 drops Benzoin
5 drops Elemi (Canarium luzonicum) EO
5 drops Myrrh (Commiphora myrrha) EO

Memory, poor
20 drops Rosemary (Rosmarinus officinalis) EO
This is good in a little mister, and you can transport this easily.

Moodiness, mood swings
You can use any with a total of twenty five drops for the blend in the 2 tablespoons carrier oil.
5 drops Eucalyptus (Eucalyptus globulus) EO
10 drops Geranium (Pelargonium graveolens) EO

10 drops Lavender (Lavendula officinalis) EO
Or
Rosewood (Aniba rosaeodora) EO
Cedarwood (Cedrus atlantica) EO
Clary Sage (Salvia sclarea) EO
Or
Coriander (Coriandrum sativum) EO
Bergamot (Citrus bergamia) EO
Peppermint (Mentha piperita) EO
Vetiver (Vetiveria zizanoides) EO

Nerves, exhausted
Nervous exhaustion is common in this day and age. We are all over-worked, over-tired and striving to get it done. These blends can help with that. We all have different nervous systems, so find a blend that will work for you.

You can use any with a total of twenty five drops for the blend in the 2 tablespoons carrier oil.
10 drops Chamomile (Matricaria chamomilla) EO
10 drops Clary Sage (Salvia sclarea) EO
5 drops Juniper (Juniperus communis) EO
Or
Lavender (Lavendula officinalis) EO
Marjoram (Origanum majorana) EO
Rosemary (Rosmarinus officinalis) EO
Black Pepper (Piper nigrum) EO
Or
Peppermint (Mentha piperita) EO
Cardamom (Elettaria cardamomum)
Rosemary (Rosmarinus officinalis) EO
Vetiver (Vetiveria zizanoides) EO
Or
15 drops Basil (Ocimum basilicum) EO
10 drops Pine (Pinus sylvestris) EO
Or
5 drops Pine (Pinus sylvestris) EO
10 drops Rosemary (Rosmarinus officinalis) EO
10 drops Clary Sage (Salvia sclarea) EO

Or
10 drops Peppermint (Mentha piperita) EO
15 drops Lavender (Lavandula angustifolia) EO
Or
5 drops Chamomile EO
10 drops Clary Sage (Salvia sclarea) EO
10 drops Vetiver (Vetiveria zizanoides) EO

Nerves, being nervy
15 drops Chamomile (Matricaria chamomilla) EO
10 drops Juniper (Juniperus communis) EO

Nightmares
15 drops each in a blend, in 2 ½ oz. carrier oil, massage on temples and spine. For children you can try 5 drops each in the carrier oil.
Frankincense (Boswellia carterii), Lavender (Lavandula angustifolia) essential oils.

Nostalgia, living in the past
5 drops Frankincense (Boswellia carterii) EO
10 drops Sandalwood (Santalum album) EO
10 drops Tangerine (Citrus reticulata) EO

Obsession
10 drops Clary Sage (Salvia sclarea) EO
10 drops Sandalwood (Santalum album) EO
5 drops Coriander

Obsession, with past
10 drops Frankincense (Boswellia carterii) EO
10 drops Sandalwood (Santalum album) EO

Obstinacy
10 drops Orange (Citrus sinensis) EO
10 drops Rosewood (Aniba rosaeodora) EO
5 drops Ylang-Ylang (Cananga odorata var genuina) EO

Overactive mind
10 drops Chamomile (Matricaria chamomilla) EO
10 drops Lavender (Lavendula officinalis) EO
5 drops Marjoram (Origanum majorana) EO

Overburdened
15 drops Rosewood (Aniba rosaeodora) EO
10 drops Sandalwood (Santalum album) EO

Overburdened, by responsibilities
15 drops Rosemary (Rosmarinus officinalis) EO
Over-emotional
10 drops Eucalyptus (Eucalyptus globulus) EO
10 drops Ravensara (Ravensara aromatica) EO

Over- talkativeness
15 drops Cypress (Cupressus sempervirens) EO

Overwork
10 drops Lavender (Lavendula officinalis) EO
15 drops Rosewood (Rosa damascena) EO

Overwork, mental strain from
We all suffer from this at times. It is a balance if being chilled out and stimulated at the same time.
10 drops Clary-sage (Salvia sclarea) EO
15 drops Rosemary (Rosmarinus officinalis) EO

Panic attacks
20 drops of the complete mixture in carrier oil.
10 drops Clary Sage (Salvia sclarea)
5 drops Frankincense (Boswellia carterii) EO
5 drops Lavender (Lavendula officinalis) EO
Or
5 drops Ylang-Ylang (Cananga odorata var genuina) EO
5 drops Chamomile (Matricaria chamomilla) EO
5 drops Spikenard (Nardostachus jatamansi) or Vetiver (Vetiveria zizanoides) EO

5 drops Rose (Rosa damascena) EO

Paranoia
10 drops Frankincense (Boswellia carterii) EO
10 drops Lavender (Lavendula officinalis) EO

Perseverance, lack of
15 drops Frankincense (Boswellia carterii) EO

Perseverance- to be able to have
10 drops Lavender (Lavandula angustifolia) EO
5 drops Sweet Orange (Citrus sinensis) EO
5 drops Rosemary (Rosmarinus officinalis) EO

Procrastination
15 drops Sandalwood (Santalum album) EO

Resentment
Releasing resentment is really hard, we all struggle with these feelings. This blend is very helpful for this issue.
Make a blend with 20-25 drops of any of the oils below.
10 drops Clary Sage (Salvia sclarea) EO
10 drops Lemon (Citrus limon) EO
Or
10 drops Sandalwood (Santalum album) EO
5 drops Ylang-Ylang (Cananga odorata var genuina) EO
5 drops Helichrysum (Helichrysum angustifolia) EO
5 drops Rose (Rosa damascena) EO

Resentment with Anger
10 drops Grapefruit (Citrus paradisi) EO
10 drops Spikenard (Nardostachys jatamansi) EO
Or
10 drops Yarrow (Achillea millefolium) EO
10 drops Yuzu (Citrus junos) EO

Resignation
15 drops Orange (Citrus sinensis) EO

5 drops Sandalwood (Santalum album) EO

Restlessness
Blend of any of the oils below, keeping it under 30 drops for 2 ½ tablespoons carrier oil.
10 drops Marjoram (Origanum majorana) EO
10 drops Frankincense (Boswellia carterii) EO
10 drops Clary Sage (Salvia sclarea) EO

Restlessness with Anxiety
10 drops Spikenard (Nardostachus jatamansi) EO
5 drops Lavender (Lavendula officinalis) EO
5 drops Vetiver (Vetiveria zizanoides) EO
5 drops Neroli (Citrus aurantium) EO
Or
10 drops Myrrh (Commiphora myrrha) EO
10 drops Vetiver (Vetiveria zizanoides) EO
5 drops Sweet Orange (Citrus sinensis) EO

Rigidity, mental
10 drops Geranium (Pelargonium graveolens) EO
15 drops Rosewood (Aniba rosaeodora) EO

Sadness
10 drops Marjoram (Origanum majorana) EO
10 drops Orange (Citrus sinensis) EO
5 drops Mandarin (Citrus reticulata) EO
Or
10 drops Juniper (Juniperus communis) EO
10 drops Grapefruit (Citrus paradisi) EO
5 drops Coriander (Mentha arvensis) EO
Or
5 drops Rosemary (Rosmarinus officinalis) EO
5 drops Bergamot (Citrus bergamia) EO
5 drops Cypress (Cupressus sempervirens) EO
5 drops Pine (Pinus sylvestris) EO

Sadness with Depression
10 drops Juniper EO
10 drops Sweet Orange (Citrus sinensis) EO
10 drops Bergamot (Citrus bergamia) EO

Selfishness, self-centeredness
10 drops Lemon (Citrus limon) EO
10 drops Orange (Citrus sinensis) EO
5 drops Sandalwood (Santalum album) EO

Self-criticism
With self-criticism all I can say is, Stop. Stop letting the voice in your head make your decisions. You are amazing just the way you are.
10 drops Frankincense (Boswellia carterii) EO
5 drops Tea Tree (Melaleuca alternifolia) EO

Self-esteem, lack of- a blend of any of these oils.
These can be helpful to have in the car on the way to a job interview, before an important meeting or before a big performance.
10 drops Juniper (Juniperus communis) EO
10 drops Sandalwood (Santalum album) EO
10 drops Ylang-Ylang (Cananga odorata var genuina) EO
Or
10 drops Rosemary (Rosmarinus officinalis) EO
10 drops Ylang-Ylang (Cananga odorata var genuina) EO
10 drops Cedarwood (Cedrus atlantica) EO
10 drops Laurel Laurus nobilis) EO
10 drops Grapefruit (Citrus paradisi) EO
Or
10 drops Jasmine (Jasminum grandiflorum) EO
10 drops Ginger (Zingiber officinale) EO
10 drops Basil (Ocimum basilicum) EO
Or
10 drops Juniper EO
10 drops Sandalwood (Santalum album) EO
10 drops Jasmine (Jasminum grandiflorum) EO

Sensitivity
10 drops Lemon (Citrus Limon) EO
10 drops Sandalwood (Santalum album) EO
5 drops Ylang-Ylang (Cananga odorata var genuina) EO
Or
10 drops Grapefruit (Citrus paradisi) EO
10 drops Sandalwood (Santalum album) EO

Shock
15 drops Tea Tree (Melaleuca alternifolia) EO
15 drops Ylang-Ylang (Cananga odorata var genuina) EO

Shyness
20 drops Spearmint (Mentha spicata) EO
10 drops Ylang-Ylang (Cananga odorata var genuina) EO
Or
10 drops Spearmint EO
10 drops Sweet Orange (Citrus sinensis) EO

Stability, need for
10 drops Frankincense (Boswellia carterii) EO
10 drops Patchouli (Pogostemon cablin) EO

Strain, mental
10 drops Chamomile (Matricaria chamomilla) EO
10 drops Clary Sage (Salvia sclarea) EO
5 drops Marjoram (Origanum majorana) EO
5 drops Rosemary (Rosmarinus officinalis) EO

Stress, general- use any of the following essential oils
Just make your blend with a total of thirty drops in your carrier oil.
Cedarwood (Cedrus atlantica), Chamomile (Matricaria chamomilla), Clary Sage (Salvia sclarea), Geranium (Pelargonium graveolens), Juniper (Juniperus communis), Lavender (Lavendula officinalis), Marjoram (Origanum majorana), Tangerine (Citrus reticulata)

Stress 1- 20 drops Tangerine (Citrus reticulata), 10 drops Lavender
Stress 2- 10 drops Marjoram, 10 drops Juniper, 10 drops Cedarwood

Stress 3- 10 drops Geranium, 10 drops Clary Sage, 10 drops Chamomile
Stress 4- 5 drops Marjoram, 20 drops Lavender, 5 drops Tangerine (Citrus reticulata)

Sulkiness
Clary Sage (Salvia sclarea), Rosewood (Aniba rosaeodora) EO
10-15 drops EO per 2 tablespoons carrier oil.

Suspiciousness
15 drops Ylang-Ylang (Cananga odorata var genuina) EO
5 drops Patchouli (Pogostemon cablin) EO

Tantrums in children
10 drops Chamomile (Matricaria chamomilla) EO
Or
10 drops Helichrysum (Helichrysum angustifolia) EO
Or
10 drops Mandarin (Citrus reticulata) EO

Tension, nervous
30 drops total of essential oil in 2 oz. of carrier oil. Any of these would work well. Add the essential oils to the carrier oil and swish the lidded bottle around, to mix the blend.
Cedarwood (Cedrus atlantica), Chamomile (Matricaria chamomilla), Clary Sage Salvia sclarea), Cypress (Cupressus sempervirens), Frankincense (Boswellia carterii), Geranium (Pelargonium graveolens), Juniper (Juniperus communis), Lavender (Lavendula officinalis), Rosewood (Aniba rosaeodora), Sandalwood (Santalum album), Tangerine (Citrus reticulata), Ylang-Ylang (Cananga odorata var genuina)

Tension 1- 10 drops Cedarwood, 10 drops Tangerine, 10 drops Sandalwood
Tension 2- 10 drops Lavender, 10 drops Clary Sage, 10 drops Chamomile
Tension 3- 10 drops Rosewood, 10 drops Sandalwood, 10 drops Frankincense.

Thoughts, gloomy
10 drops Orange (Citrus sinensis) EO
20 drops Mandarin (Citrus reticulata) EO

Thoughts, irrational
10 drops Marjoram (Origanum majorana) EO
5 drops Grapefruit (Citrus paradisi) EO
5 drops Tea Tree (Melaleuca alternifolia) EO

Thoughts, negative
15 drops Clary Sage (Salvia sclarea) EO
15 drops Lavender (Lavendula officinalis) EO

Thoughts, racing
15 drops Clary Sage (Salvia sclarea) EO
10 drops Neroli (Citrus aurantium) EO

Thoughts, restless
20 drops Chamomile (Matricaria chamomilla) EO
5 drops Clary Sage (Salvia sclarea) EO

Thoughts, scattered
15 drops Cedarwood (Cedrus atlantica) EO
5 drops Grapefruit (Citrus paradisi) EO

Thoughts, unclear
15 drops Eucalyptus (Eucalyptus globulus) EO
15 drops Grapefruit (Citrus paradisi) EO
Or
10 drops Lemon (Citrus limon) EO
10 drops Peppermint (Mentha piperita) EO
10 drops Rosemary (Rosmarinus officinalis) EO

Touchiness
15 drops Lemon (Citrus limon) EO
10 drops Mandarin (Citrus reticulata) or Grapefruit (Citrus paradisi) EO

Uncleanness, feelings of
15 drops Tea Tree (Melaleuca alternifolia) EO
5 drops Rosemary (Rosmarinus officinalis) or Ravensara (Ravensara aromatica)
EO

Unable to Forgive

Being unable to forgive hurts you more than the person you are unable to forgive.

15 drops Sandalwood (Santalum album) EO

15 drops Patchouli (Pogostemon cablin) EO

Unable to Forgive- Learning to let go

15 drops Sandalwood (Santalum album) EO

10 drops Sweet Orange (Citrus sinensis) EO

10 drops Clary Sage (Salvia sclarea) EO

Unyielding to circumstances

10 drops Rosewood (Aniba rosaeodora) EO

10 drops Patchouli (Pogostemon cablin) EO

Weak-willed

15 drops Cypress (Cupressus sempervirens) EO

5 drops Patchouli (Pogostemon cablin) EO

Withdrawnness

Being withdrawn can be worrisome and tiresome for the sufferer. A few sprays of this can assist with these feelings.

10 drops Marjoram (Origanum majorana) EO

5 drops Ravensara (Ravensara aromatica) EO

Worry

15 drops Chamomile (Matricaria chamomilla) EO

10 drops Juniper (Juniperus communis) EO

Worry, about future

10 drops Lavender (Lavendula officinalis) EO

Body Wash? Yes, if you want to add any of these blends to a body wash you can do the following:

Make a body wash out of Castile Soap, unscented and add the essential oil blends to at least 6 ounces of body wash. Mix well and use in the shower.

Purchase an unscented body wash base. Add the essential oil blend to at least 6 ounces of body wash, mix well and use as directed.

10 drops Sandalwood (Santalum album) EO
5 drops Clary-Sage (Salvia sclarea) EO

Worry, about past
10 drops Frankincense (Boswellia carterii) EO
5 drops Mandarin (Citrus reticulata) EO

Mists that are helpful in Labor and Delivery
Nausea Spray
Add the following to four ounces of distilled water and use in a spray bottle:
20 drops Spearmint (Mentha spicata) EO
15 drops Lemon EO
5 drops Sweet Orange (Citrus sinensis) EO
Shake the mixture well and mist the air with it when a woman feels nauseous. You may find that different women prefer other types of scents, so you can also try Ginger (Zingiber officinale), Neroli (Citrus aurantium) and Rosewood. Experiment to find the mixture that works best. When making an alternative blend, keep the amount of essential oils used at less than 60 drops.
This works for morning sickness, nausea in transition, motion sickness and overall nausea.

Labor Mists
The point of using mists during labor is to be as noninvasive as possible. Every person is different and has individual needs. Make sure that you understand and know the person you are making a blend for because the wrong blend can assault the senses. In our need to help, we do not want to create something not so beautiful for a mother.

Relax and Focus
This is a relaxing blend to promote clarity and focus. Fill a four-ounce spray bottle almost full with distilled water and add:
20 drops Grapefruit (Citrus paradisi) essential oil
15 drops Sweet Orange (Citrus sinensis) essential oil
10 drops Spearmint essential oil
Shake well and mist labor room. You can also make a compress by misting a wet cloth with the blend and applying it to the laboring mother's forehead or back. This mist is great for fathers, too.

Uplift

Transition can be a trying and tiring time for the mother. We want to support her and use a mist blend that will ground and calm her and help lift her spirits. Add water to spray bottle as above and add:

15 drops Mandarin essential oil

10 drops Bergamot (Citrus bergamia) essential oil

10 drops Lavender (Lavandula angustifolia) essential oil

10 drops Clary Sage (Salvia sclarea) essential oil

This is a strong blend and it should be used away from the mother. Never spray the mother directly.

Always remember to use essential oils with education and care. Research each oil before use, especially in regard to pregnancy and labor.

Make sure when you are using a mist in an environment like a birth you that you make sure any scent can be taken away. So misting a pillow, washcloth or compress are all ways you can work with the oils, but make sure it can be removed if the scent becomes offensive.

Urinating After Birth

If a mother is having a hard time urinating after birth a few drops of peppermint oil in the toilet bowl usually is of assistance.

Demetria Clark

5 SALVES, OINTMENTS, BALMS AND LINIMENTS AND MUCH MORE...

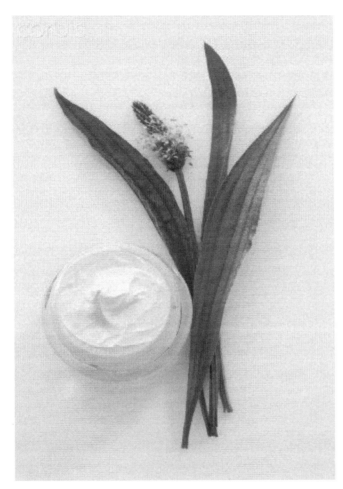

Salve, Balms and Ointments are essentially fats and waxes being used to carry herbal medicine to the skin, and other topical issues.

Some tips for making salves Infuse your oils beforehand, so you have them on hand when you are making salves and you won't be tempted to take short cuts. An infused oil that is strained and decanted into a sterile jar will last for about a year, made into a salve it will last for many years. You can also freeze the infused oils in a freezer safe jar. Give the oil room to expand. When thawing remove the lid and gently warm in a double boiler to insure proper thawing, and that no ice crystal are becoming water in the oil.

If you salve is too hard, then you can re-melt and add a little more oil. You can place a small amount of the salve in the freezer for a few minutes to test hardness.

If your salve is too soft, you can re-melt it and add a little more beeswax. You will find eventually you will be able to tell from texture if you need more or less wax.

Using hard oils like coconut, mango butter, Shea butter and cocoa butter will change wax ratios.

Wax amounts cannot be exact. Oil thicknesses, humidity and types of waxes used will change the consistency of your salve, balm or ointment.

Some beeswax tips, these will come in handy when a recipe is listed as parts, instead of exact measurements. One pint of oil will need about 1 ½-2 ounces of beeswax, or one ounce of oil will need about 1/2 teaspoon of beeswax. Approximately 5 teaspoons of beeswax is in an ounce. Shredding beeswax will make it melt in faster and easier. You can also buy beeswax in pastilles also.

Invest in some salve pots, small jars, or small containers. It is good to have some on hand for storing salves. This way you can have them on hand in case you have an oil ready and you are interested in making a salve. You find double walled jars online, or a bottle company. Some use small jam jars, baby food jars, or ceramic pots. Two to four ounce sizes seem to work the best.

What are balms and ointments?
In my definition a balm is a softer salve, and an ointment is almost runny. If you go to a pharmacy you will usually find ointments in tubes, like hemorrhoid treatments. Even though they have lost a little in popularity, I really love ointments, personally. I like that they can be put in a transportable tube and can be easily made.

Skin Issue Salves
Cracked Skin Salve
2 oz. Beeswax
2 oz. Calendula (Calendula officinalis) infused olive oil
2 oz. Plantain (Plantago major) infused olive oil
2 oz. St. John's Wort (Hypericum perforatum) infused olive oil
Melt all together until beeswax is melted then add:
12 drops Vitamin E
12 drops Pine needle EO
10 drops Chamomile (German) EO
12 drops Lavender (Lavandula angustifolia) EO
10 drops Tea Tree (Melaleuca alternifolia) EO.
Warm the oil and melt in the shredded beeswax, stir in to melt, remove from the heat and add the essential oils, stir. Pour into jars or tubs, and allow it to set. Cool

a bit, then pour into clean jars.

Black Walnut Salve

This salve is helpful for ringworm and fungal infections.

2 part Black Walnut

2 part Chaparral

2 part Myrrh (Commiphora myrrha)

1 part Burdock Root

Infuse all of the herbs in Olive Oil for 3-6 weeks.

You will need 2 cups of oil for the recipe, so if want add the herbs to 2 cups of olive oil. Strain well.

You will want to warm the oil and add to it:

2 oz. Beeswax

20 drops Vitamin E

Tea Tree (Melaleuca alternifolia) Oil - 60 drops essential oil for 2 cups of oil.

Warm the oil and melt in the shredded beeswax, stir in to melt, remove from the heat and add the essential oils, stir. Pour into jars or tubs, and allow it to set.

Goldenseal Calendula Salve

3 oz. Olive Oil infused with Calendula (Calendula officinalis) Flowers

2 oz. Olive Oil infused with Goldenseal Powder/Chopped Root

2 oz. Olive Oil infused with Plantain Leaf

3 oz. shredded beeswax

30 drops of Tea Tree (Melaleuca alternifolia) EO

40 drops of Lavender (Lavandula angustifolia) EO

1/8 teaspoon Vitamin E oil

This salve is for infections, yeast issues and

Yarrow Salve

2 cups Yarrow infused oil (Achillea millefolium)

¼ cup shredded Beeswax lightly packed

Warm the oil and melt in the shredded beeswax, stir in to melt. Pour into jars or tubs, and allow it to set. This can be helpful for cuts, scrapes and conditions asking for a more astringent salve or balm.

Plantain Salve

2 cups Plantain infused oil (Plantago major)

¼ cup shredded Beeswax lightly packed

Warm the oil and melt in the shredded beeswax, stir in to melt. Pour into jars or tubs, and allow it to set. This can be helpful for cuts, scrapes and stings. I love using this on reactions from stinging nettle plants.

St. John's Wort Salve
2 cups St. John's Wort (Hypericum perforatum) infused oil
¼ cup shredded Beeswax lightly packed
Warm the oil and melt in the shredded beeswax, stir in to melt. Pour into jars or tubs, and allow it to set. This salve is helpful for irritated rough skin.

Soothing Salve Recipe© Demetria Clark
Use oil infused with one part of each plant
Plantain (Plantago major)
Comfrey (Symphytum officinale)
St. John's Wort (Hypericum perforatum)
Calendula (Calendula officinalis)
Then add an essential oil such as Lavender (Lavandula angustifolia) or Tea Tree (Melaleuca alternifolia) oil. Add only a few drops, use essential oil sparingly it is very potent.

Great Gardener Salve
1 part whole Calendula (Calendula officinalis) flowers infused in oil.
1-part meadowsweet (Filipendula ulmaria) flowers, buds and leaves infused in oil.
1 part Plantain (Plantago major) Leaf infused oil.
This one is good for gardeners; the Meadowsweet eases the muscle ache and the Calendula helps with the rough skin, Plantain soothes the skin. Make into a salve following previous directions.

Salves For What is Underneath
Nerve Pain Salve
1 cup St. John's Wort (Hypericum perforatum) infused oil
1 cup Devil's Claw (Harpagophytum procumbens)
¼ cup shredded Beeswax lightly packed
20 drops of Lavender (Lavandula angustifolia) EO
10 drops Marjoram EO
Warm the oil and melt in the shredded beeswax, stir in to melt. Pour into jars or tubs, and allow it to set Massage into the area that is in pain.

Sciatica Salve

1 cup Black Cohosh Root infused oil- Black Cohosh is a wonderful topical treatment for sciatic pain, and it makes a wonderful liniment also.

1 cup St. John's Wort (Hypericum perforatum) infused Oil.

¼cup shredded Beeswax lightly packed

20 drops of Lavender (Lavandula angustifolia) EO

10 drops Peppermint (Mentha piperita) EO

Warm the oil and melt in the shredded beeswax, stir in to melt. Pour into jars or tubs, and allow it to set.

Use on where your sciatic pain is coming from. Make sure you also massage into the surrounding tissue to support the nerve.

Sciatica Oil- *Make the salve above, but leave out the beeswax and use as an oil, apply to the affected area.*

Sore Muscle Salve

1/4 cup Arnica (Arnica montana) infused oil

1/4 cup Devil's Claw infused oil

1/4 cup St. John's Wort (Hypericum perforatum) infused oil

1/4 cup Chamomile infused oil

1/4 cup Beeswax

10 drops of each essential oils: Juniper, Spearmint, Rosemary (Rosmarinus officinalis), Ginger (Zingiber officinale), Eucalyptus and Lime

Warm the oil and melt in the shredded beeswax, stir in to melt. Add the essential oils, stir well. Pour into jars or tubs, and allow it to set.

Use on sore muscles.

Cayenne Muscle Salve

Cayenne Infused oil- in one cup of oil add ¼ cup cayenne powder. Warm the oil in a double boiler and stir in the cayenne. Allow it to remain in the double boiler on low heat for a half hour, then remove from the stove. Allow the oil too steep for another 24 hours lightly covered. Strain through cheese cloth, or a fine linen cloth.

After you have strained the oil warm it and add to it ¼ cup beeswax and 1 teaspoon Vitamin E.

Pour into jars and allow to set.

To use, patch test first. This can be really potent and everyone reacts differently. Make sure the salve does irritate your skin.

Shoulder Tension Salve
¼ cup Arnica (Arnica montana) infused Oil
¼ cup Lavender (Lavandula angustifolia) Infused Oil
½ cup Calendula (Calendula officinalis) Infused Oil
10 drops Lavender (Lavandula angustifolia)
Warm the oil and melt in the shredded beeswax, stir in to melt. Add the essential oils, stir well. Pour into jars or tubs, and allow it to set.
Use on stir and sore shoulder.

Camphor Wowzer Balm
This is a really strong balm. Great for sore muscles.
2 oz. beeswax shredded
1/2 cup olive oil
Warm the oil, over low heat, and add the beeswax until melted.
Remove from heat. Then add the essential oil, stir and pour into your containers.
20 drops camphor essential oil
12 drops Peppermint (Mentha piperita) essential oil
12 drops eucalyptus essential oil
10 drops clove essential oil
10 drops cinnamon essential oil
This is good for acute and tension related pain.

Varicose Vein Salve
1 part Calendula (Calendula officinalis) infused oil
1 part horse chestnut (Aesculus hippocastanum) bark, leaf, and/or green chopped-up fruit –infused in oil
2 parts St. John's Wort (Hypericum perforatum) infused oil.
Make into a salve.

Stretch Mark Balm
1/2 cup cocoa butter
2 Tablespoons wheat germ oil
2 teaspoons Sesame seed oil

2 teaspoon Rose hip seed oil
2 teaspoons Vitamin E oil
4 teaspoons grated beeswax
1 teaspoon Lavender (Lavandula angustifolia), Sandalwood (Santalum album), Palmarosa or Neroli (Citrus aurantium) essential oil.
Gentle heat the cocoa butter and beeswax until they have melted; stir well, add the other oils. Remove from the heat and stir in the essential oil of choice. Pour into a clean jar or container, and allow to cool.

Callous Balm

3/4 cup olive oil
1/2 cup avocado oil
3 tablespoons jojoba oil
1 teaspoon vitamin E oil
2 oz. beeswax, you can add more if you want a harder balm
12 drops Lavender (Lavandula angustifolia) EO
12 drops Rosemary (Rosmarinus officinalis) EO
10 drops Lemon or Sweet Orange (Citrus sinensis) EO
Heat the oils, and melt beeswax into the warming oil. When the beeswax is melted allow the oils to cool for a few minutes and then add the essential oils, pour into clean jars of pots.

Lion Balm

3 tablespoons Camphor Oil EO
3 tablespoons Eucalyptus EO
3 tablespoons Lavender (Lavandula angustifolia) EO
5 tablespoons Peppermint (Mentha piperita) EO
4 tablespoons Wintergreen EO
1/2 cup Jojoba Oil
1/4 cup grated beeswax
Warm the Jojoba and melt the beeswax, when the beeswax is cooling add the essential oil and pour into clean jars.

Congestion Balm

½ cup olive oil
½ cup coconut oil
¼ cup shredded beeswax
20 drops of Eucalyptus EO

20 drops Peppermint (Mentha piperita) EO
10 drops Tea Tree (Melaleuca alternifolia) EO
10 drops Lavender (Lavandula angustifolia) EO
Warm the oil and melt the shredded beeswax into the warming oil. Once the beeswax is melted remove from heat, allow to cool for a few minutes, add the essential oils and stir in gently. Pour into clean jars of pots.

For Babies
Natural Diaper Rash Balm
This natural blend will soothe the skin, heal and calm any inflammations. Apply directly to affected area.
1 oz. Calendula (Calendula officinalis) infused olive oil
1/2 oz. Avocado oil
1/2 oz. Coconut oil
2 drops of Lavender (Lavandula angustifolia) essential oil
Warm the coconut oil and melt, add the infused Calendula and avocado oil, stir well.
Stir in two drops of lavender essential oil. Pour into a 2 oz. jar. Allow to cool before use.

Cradle Cap blend
In 4 oz. Olive oil infuse Calendula (Calendula officinalis) flower and Chamomile flower.
Cradle cap is a fact of life. It is when the oily scalp of baby causes a "pile up" of excess skin that becomes flaky and crusty. Do not pick. Apply an oil and gently comb the scalp and hair, use a cotton ball in the eyebrows and behind ears if it is present there. Wash head gently. Use a nice olive oil. Do not use mineral oil.
Or
At night apply the olive oil and allow it to stay on baby's head until morning. Comb out and wash in the morning.
Or
You can slough off the oily scalp and oil with a very soft toothbrush.

LINIMENTS and LINIMENT OILS

A liniment is an herbal extraction in a liquid, such as alcohol, oil, or vinegar, which is rubbed into the skin to treat arthritis, inflammations, sore muscles, and strains.

LINIMENT OIL

Essentially a liniment oil, is an infused oil. But because I am using them like I would a traditional liniment, I am calling them liniment oils. These recipes would also be at home in the infused oil section.

To make one of my favorite liniments, place four ounces each fresh or dried Peppermint (Mentha piperita) and eucalyptus leaves in a 16-ounce jar.
Cover with a pint of vodka or vinegar. (Do not use rubbing alcohol.)
Personally I really like vodka for my liniments, it has very little scent once applied, extracts plant constituents well and has a very long shelf life. Vinegar is good also, but I thought I would share my preference.

Let the mixture set in a dry place for fourteen days and shake the contents twice a day. (You can also add a few drops of essential oil, such as eucalyptus, Peppermint (Mentha piperita), or Rosemary (Rosmarinus officinalis), if you like.)

For an "instant" liniment, mix one teaspoon of essential oil of peppermint, eucalyptus, or rosemary with one-half cup of vodka.

Some of my favorite herbs to use in liniments are:
Sweet Clover (Melilotus officinalis) – is a great herb for nerve pain.

Goldenrod (Solidago altissima) – Wonderful for muscle trauma, pain and injuries. This is a great herb for athletes in a liniment, we have used it for skateboarding, football and dancing injuries.

Comfrey (Symphytum officinale) -Divine for any kind of swelling, bruising, blunt trauma kind of thing as well as broken bones.

Peppermint (Mentha piperita) or Spearmint (Mentha spicata)- cooling pain relief.

St. John's Wort (Hypericum perforatum) flowers- excellent for muscle and nerve pain.

Ginger (Zingiber officinale)- warming liniment, for muscular pain.

Rosemary- A strong pain relieving herb.

Black Pepper (Piper nigrum)- Strong pain relieving herb.

Liniment Base
2 cups Vodka or vinegar
Cover 1 cup of ripped Peppermint (Mentha piperita) leaf.
Allow this to sit for two to four weeks and add your essential oils.

Sore Muscle Liniment
2 cups vodka or cider vinegar
1 cup chopped St. John's Wort (Hypericum perforatum) flowers and leaves
Allow this to sit for two to four weeks and add your essential oils.
20 drops Black Pepper (Piper nigrum) Essential oil
20 drops Lavender (Lavandula angustifolia) Essential oil
Mix well and apply to sore muscles.

When applying a liniment apply in a massage like fashion. This allows it to penetrate the muscles and tissues, so you can really feel it and get the benefit of it.

My Favorite Football Liniment

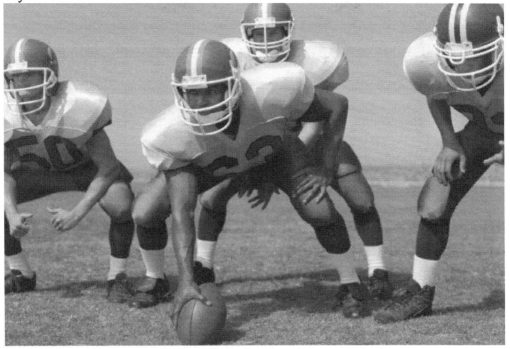

1 part Comfrey (Symphytum officinale) dried or fresh herb
1 part St. John's Wort (Hypericum perforatum) dried or fresh herb.
1 part Goldenrod dried or fresh herb
Place dried herb in a jar and cover with vodka or cider vinegar.
After it has sat for 4 weeks add a few drops Black Pepper (Piper nigrum) and
Lavender essential oil.

Arnica Liniment

Arnica (Arnica montana) liniment should not be used on broken skin, but it is
excellent for bruising, welts, etc... Recently studies have suggested it may also be
helpful in the management of burns.

Arnica has been used medicinally since the 1500s. Arnica is used topically for
a wide range of disorders, to include bruising, sprains, muscle aches, wound
healing, joint pain, inflammation from insect bites, and swelling from broken
bones.

Fill a glass jar with Arnica (Arnica montana) flowers
Cover with vodka and allow it to sit for 2 months.
Shake slightly every day. Strain and decant for use.

Arnica Liniment II

1 part Arnica (Arnica montana) Flower
1 part St. John's Wort (Hypericum perforatum) flower
Put in a jar and cover with vodka, cover.
Allow it to sit for 2 months and shake slightly every day.
Strain and decant for use.

Arnica Infused Oil

Fill a jar with Arnica (Arnica montana) Flowers, cover with olive oil. Allow it to infuse for at least two weeks. Strain and decant.
Use as you would with the liniment.

Arnica SJW Oil

1 part Arnica (Arnica montana) flower
1 part St. John's Wort (Hypericum perforatum) Flower
Place the flowers in a canning jar cover with olive oil.
Allow the oil to steep covered for 3-6 weeks.
Shake lightly every day. Strain and decant for use.

Arnica Calendula Liniment

1 part Arnica (Arnica montana) flower
1 part Calendula (Calendula officinalis) flower
Place the flowers in a canning jar cover with vodka.
Allow the mixture to steep covered for 3-6 weeks.
Shake lightly every day. Strain and decant for use.

Arnica Calendula Oil

1 part Arnica flower
1 part Calendula (Calendula officinalis) flower
Place the flowers in a canning jar cover with olive oil.
Allow the oil to steep covered for 3-6 weeks.
Shake lightly every day. Strain and decant for use. This is so helpful for sore muscles and strains.

Calendula St. St. John's Wort Oil

2 parts Calendula (Calendula officinalis) Flower
1 part St. John's Wort (Hypericum perforatum) Flower
Place the flowers in a canning jar cover with vodka.

Allow the mixture to steep covered for 3-6 weeks.

Shake lightly every day. Strain and decant for use.

This is wonderful for nerve pain, sore muscles and stressed muscles.

Calendula St. John's Wort Peppermint Oil

1 part Calendula (Calendula officinalis) Flower

1 part St. John's Wort (Hypericum perforatum) Flower

1 part Peppermint Herb

Place the flowers in a canning jar cover with olive oil.

Allow the oil to steep covered for 3-6 weeks.

Shake lightly every day. Strain and decant for use.

This is also good for nerve and muscle pain, but the peppermint adds an extra strength to the oil.

Ginger Liniment

1 part shredded Ginger root. I like to use a piece the size of my palm, and add it to a quart canning jar.

Place the flowers in a canning jar cover with vodka.

Allow the mixture to steep covered for 3-6 weeks.

Shake lightly every day. Strain and decant for use.

Make sure it is not too strong before you use it. Dilute with water or vodka as needed when used. Do not pre-dilute, dilute when needed.

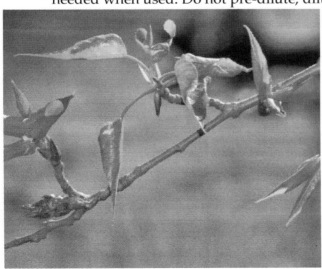

Cottonwood Liniment

2 parts Cottonwood buds

1 part Sweet Clover

1 part Ginger Root Shredded

½ part Calendula (Calendula officinalis) flower

Place the flowers in a canning jar cover with vodka.

Allow the mixture to steep covered for 3-6 weeks.

Shake lightly every day. Strain and decant for use.

Witch Hazel Liniment

Witch hazel (Hamamelis virginiana) serves as a base for many remedies for varicose veins, vaginal area varicosities and hemorrhoids.

1 cup 80 proof alcohol, 1 cup water, 1 cup witch hazel leaves *(Hamamelis virginiana)*

Cover the leaves with the alcohol and water. You can add more leaves if you want. After four weeks strain and bottle. Add five to ten drops Cypress (Cupressus sempervirens) oil, if desired. Apply to affected area with a cool cloth.

Hemorrhoid Liniment

Apply the following herbal teas, once cooled, to the area: St. John's Wort, Witch-hazel (Hamamelis virginiana), plantain leaf (Plantago major), sage (Salvia off.), Parsley (Petroselinum crispum), shepherd's purse (Capsella bursa-pastoris).

Create afterwipes by applying witch hazel extract (Hamamelis virginiana) to soft small flannel clothes, cotton pads or soft toilet paper. The flannels can be washed and remade. These can also be used for tears and swelling. Cotton pads from the drug store placed in a small plastic food container and covered with witch hazel extract (Hamamelis virginiana) also make wonderful healing wipes for a woman after birth.

Athletes Foot Vinegar Liniment

1-pint organic cider vinegar
1 teaspoon Lavender flower
1-teaspoon Oregano
Allow it to macerate for 2 weeks.

You can make a healing salve from Comfrey, Calendula (Calendula officinalis) and Plantain (Plantago major). This would be soothing and beneficial for rare dry

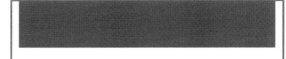

Powders for Fungal Issues

Athletes Foot Powder
1 part Cornstarch
2 parts Arrowroot powder
1 part ground Calendula
1/2 part ground Myrrh

Sprinkle on the inflamed or irritated area. You can also soak your tea feet in a calendula and myrrh tea. Add two cups of tea to a foot bath.

Jock Itch Powder
1 part Arrowroot
1 part Corn Starch
¼ part Myrrh
1/8 part ground Goldenseal root. Ground to a fine powder.

A drop or two of tea tree essential oil. Allow the mixture to sit for 3-4 days before using, shake once a day. Sprinkle on affected area.
You can also use ground thyme, sage, and oregano and thyme or peppermint essential oil.

feet.

Fungal Infection Liniment

1 pint organic apple cider vinegar

1 tablespoon oregano

1 tablespoon Calendula (Calendula officinalis) flower

Allow to macerate for 2 weeks. Add 10 drops Tea Tree (Melaleuca alternifolia) Essential oil.

Apply on areas affected by fungal issues. It can also be applied as a compress.

Rinses

Yeast Rinse

This rinse can assist with yeasty skin issues like diaper rash, thrush or Tinea. Yeast rashes can be painful, ooze or sticky feeling. It is important to keep the area clean and dry. You can find the affliction in skin creases, the groin, skin folds, hairline, mouth and genitals, so make sure you treat all areas with issues.

2 tablespoons acidophilus powder

2 cups Sage Tea

2 drops Tea Tree (Melaleuca alternifolia) Essential oil.

Pour over the affected area or apply with a cloth on the inflamed area.

Psoriasis Relief Rinse

Fill a quart jar with Dandelion (Taraxacum officinale) and Nettles (Urtica dioica)

Pinch powdered Cayenne pepper

Cover with Organic Apple Cider Vinegar

Allow it to infuse for 3 weeks, strain and rebottle.

Make sure you use an airtight containers for storage.

Add 20 drops of Peppermint (Mentha piperita) Essential oil per 1 cup of rinse.

Apply to the affected area.

Shingles Rinse

Shingles can be incredibly painful. I have heard many people claim that shingles was the worst pain they had ever experienced. Rinses can be a beneficial part of the healing process. Many people experience the pain and exhaustion for much longer than they are told they will. Allow your body the time it needs to heal.

1 cup Listerine Mouth Wash (Listerine contains the following essential oils, eucalyptol (the chief constituent of eucalyptus oil), menthol (from the Mint

family), methyl salicylate (menthol), and thymol (constituent in Thyme).
1 cup Lemon Balm (Melissa officinalis) Tea
1 cup Oregano Tea
Use as a compress or rinse on the shingles rash.

Shingles Rinse II
1 cup Lemon Balm (Melissa officinalis) Tea
1 cup Mullein Leaf tea
1 cup Chamomile tea
Mix all three together and use as a rinse or compress.
Or make by the gallon and add them to a bath tub for a soak.
You can also make compresses from these rinses. Apply the compress and allow it to rest on the area, replacing every 20-30 minutes.

Pastes
When making a paste make sure you use powdered herb and mix it with tea, water or another liquid and make sure it is thick and stiff, like a frosting or toothpaste.
Slowly add the water to the herb and mix until you have the right consistency.

Pastes for Boils
For each add the water to herb and add to the boil site, cover with a bandage. If the boil has opened do not use the pastes on it. Make a paste from any of the single herbs listed below, or a combination of two. Do not apply on open or oozing boils, this is foreign bodies are not introduced into the boil directly. You can also make Turmeric tea and make a compress to apply on the boil directly.
Powdered Turmeric
Powdered Mustard
Powdered Comfrey
Epsom Salts (when made into a paste will make a homemade magnesium sulfate paste.)
Allow the paste to dry, and then rinse off with warm water. After apply a liquid witch hazel, or Echinacea extract to the area. This also works on chest and back acne.

Pastes for Spots
Spots are also called pimples or zits. This paste works really well, and it is especially helpful on back or shoulder acne.

1 part pink clay
1 part powdered oatmeal
1 part rose petals
Blend all together, add enough water, tea or witch hazel to make a paste.
Apply to the pimples and allow the mixture to stay on the spots for at least 20 minutes.
Allow the paste to dry, and then rinse off with warm water. After apply a liquid witch hazel extract to the area. This also works on chest and back acne.

Paste for Varicose Veins
Powdered St. John's Wort (Hypericum perforatum) Flowers
Powdered Plantain (Plantago major) Leaf
Make into a past and gently apply to area. This can assist with some of the pain associated with varicose veins. Make sure you do not apply with pressure on the veins, just paint over the veins.
Allow the paste to dry, and then rinse off with warm water. After apply a liquid witch hazel extract to the area. This also works on chest and back acne.

Paste for Tennis Elbow
Fenugreek (Trigon Ella foenum-graecum) seed, powdered, fenugreek is anti-inflammatory.
Turmeric powder is a strong anti-inflammatory and painkiller.
Use 1 part each with water and make into a paste and apply to the elbow. Leave the paste on for a ½ hour, wash off and apply Arnica Oil.
This paste can also be used on sore knees, and hips.

Paste for Bottom Acne
1 part Green Clay
1 part powdered chickweed
1 part powdered yarrow or witch hazel leaf
1 part powdered black tea
Add water and make into a paste.
Make into a paste, add one to two drops of essential oil of Tea Tree.
Apply the paste to the pimples on the buttocks. Allow the paste to dry, and then rinse off with warm water. After apply a liquid witch hazel extract to the area. This also works on chest and back acne.

Tips for Pastes

1. You can make and store them.
2. You can premix, to use while camping, have in a first aid kit or in the car. Just add water when ready.
3. Pastes can be made and put into tubes and tubs for easy storage and application.
4. You can use vegetable oil or glycerin to make the paste store in a softer application.

6 FACE AND HAIR

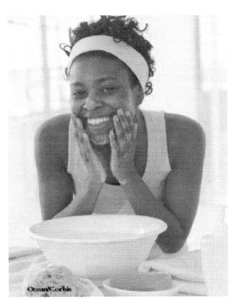

Natural skin and household cleaners are not only safer for families and the environment, but they are cheaper. So you can keep your face, body and house clean, save money and the planet, it is a win, win situation.

Scrub Your Mug Recipes
Sage Toner
1 cup Witch Hazel (Hamamelis virginiana)
½ cup Distilled Water (you can also use a floral water)
½ cup Sage infusion
1 teaspoon Aloe Vera
1 teaspoon Vegetable Glycerin (optional)
8-10 drops *Essential oil either Rosemary (Rosmarinus officinalis), Tea Tree (Melaleuca alternifolia) or Clary Sage (Salvia sclarea)
You can also add fresh Rosemary, lavender or rose to the Sage infusion.
Apply nightly with a cotton ball on the whole face and neck, behind the ears and other places of oily skin. Keep out of your eyes.

Sage Face Wash
1 cup liquid castile soap or liquid soap base
¼ cup strong Sage infusion
3 drops Clary Sage (Salvia sclarea) Essential oil
½ teaspoon Powdered pectin
Blend together and put in a pump bottle and you have a blemish fighting face wash. You can also a drop of Tea Tree (Melaleuca alternifolia) essential oil, Rosemary (Rosmarinus officinalis) or Lavender (Lavandula angustifolia) essential oil.

Acne Formulas
Acne, Blemish Remover Formula
Dried Herbs:

2 parts Red Clover (Trifolium pratense)

2 parts Dandelion (Taraxacum officinale) Root

1 part Echinacea Flower (Echinacea angustifolia)

1 part Alfalfa leaf (Medicago sativa)

1/2 part Capsicum

Add 2 tablespoons to a cup of water and allow steeping for twenty minutes. Apply as a compress, or drink as a tea. It does have capsicum, so it will be hot.

Acne Toner
1 cup apple cider vinegar

¼ cup tea made with oregano, and lavender

2 drops Rosemary Essential Oil

Apply to the pimples with cotton balls, 1-2 times a day.

Zit Zapper Toner
Infuse witch hazel as above with

1 ½ cups Witch Hazel (Hamamelis virginiana)

1 teaspoon Peppermint (Mentha piperita) leaf

1 teaspoon Sage (Salvia officinalis)

1 teaspoon Rosemary (Rosmarinus officinalis)

1 drop Camphor Essential Oil

1 drop Tea Tree (Melaleuca alternifolia) Essential Oil

3-5 drops Echinacea Extract (Echinacea angustifolia)

Allow the mixture to macerate for two days. Shake daily and when the mixture is ready strain well. Bottle and use two times a day. Shake before using. If the mixture is too strong you can add more water.

Maceration- softening by soaking in liquid, to soak, steep or marinate or saturate.

Cucumber Astringent/Tightener/Toner
Cucumber is a cooling, and gentle astringent, easy to find and it works internally as well as externally. I bet you have seen cucumbers on eyes, on television, spas, and magazine illustrations since your childhood. This is a remedy as old as time. You can use the juice or mashed pulp. It is also said that eating the vegetable or the juice can have a beneficial effect on your complexion.

Apply to face and allow it to sit on your skin for 15-20 minutes.

Lecithin Toner

Dissolve lecithin granules in jojoba or sesame oil. You can apply to face and throat as a day or night cream.

Lemon Toner

1/2 cup lemon juice
1 cup water
2/3 cup Witch hazel (Hamamelis virginiana)
10 drops Rose Essential Oil.
Combine all ingredients. Pour into a clean bottle Shake well before using. Apply with a clean cotton ball or cotton cloth. Lemon can irritate some people's skin, so patch test, as you would with any new remedy, or cosmetic.

Pine Toner

2 cups fresh white pine needles
1 cup water
1/2 cup Witch hazel (Hamamelis virginiana)
10 drops Rosemary (Rosmarinus officinalis) EO
10 drops Rose Hip Seed Oil.
Make a pine needle infusion. Allow water to cool completely then strain and discard pine needles. Add witch hazel and stir well. Pour into a clean bottle, shake well and apply to skin with a cotton ball or cotton cloth.

Queen of Hungary Water

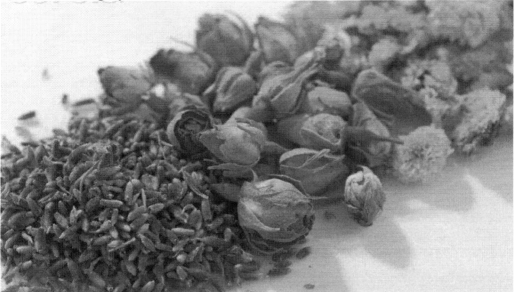

This is an ancient recipe for skin care, and has many versions and every herbalist has their own version based on the recipe of old.

Some stories of the water include it being used to reverse aging, others have it as being a heal-all water for all sorts of topical issues.

1 part Roses petals
1 part Lavender flowers
1 part Rosemary (Rosmarinus officinalis)
1 part Sage (Salvia officinalis)
1 part Comfrey (Symphytum officinale) leaf
1 part Lemon Balm (Melissa officinalis)
1 part Orange peel
1 part Lemon peel
2 parts Spearmint

Place in a jar and cover with apple cider vinegar, allow it steep in a jar for 2-3 weeks. When it is ready strain well and cut it with rosewater. So if you have 1 cup add 1 cup rosewater to it and bottle for use.

You can also alter the water by adding Calendula (Calendula officinalis), Lilac, Carnation or Hyssop flowers or a few drops of Lavender or Rose essential oils.

Antique Queen of Hungary Water

This recipe is based on the list of "old world" herbs used.

2 parts Rosemary (Rosmarinus officinalis)

1 part of the following herbs Lavender, Spearmint, Marjoram, Costus, Orange blossom and Lemon.

Cover with Brandy and allow it too steep for 4 weeks. Strain and decant.

Rose Water & Glycerin Astringent

1/2 pint olive oil

1 ounce rose water or hydrosol

A few drops of vegetable glycerin

1 ounce vodka

2 drops Rose absolute

Add all to a jar and mix well. Shaking is a good way to combine all of the ingredients.

Do It Yourself Scrub

1 part oil of choice, use almond, olive or avocado oils, they are the best.

1 part abrasive (salt, fine sand, ground oatmeal, ground almonds, etc.) I like mixing oatmeal and a little sea salt.

2 to 5 drops of essential oil of choice.

Try these oils for skin's different needs

Soothing- Lavender, Chamomile

Invigorating- Tea Tree, Peppermint (Mentha piperita)

Start off with less Essential Oil at first so you don't overdo it.

Acne- Tea Tree (Melaleuca alternifolia) oil, Patchouli (Pogostemon cablin), Geranium (Pelargonium graveolens)

Dermatitis- Hyssop, Juniper, Cedarwood (Cedrus atlantica)

Dry Skin: Cedarwood (Cedrus atlantica) - Ylang-Ylang (Cananga odorata var genuina), Rose, Rosewood and Lavender

You may also add 1 part liquid soap, or castile soap, if desired. This just gives it suds and a smoother texture.

Mix well with a fork. Apply gently to skin and shower or bath as usual.

Goddess Face Scrub
Combine together in a bowl:
1 cup of finely ground dried Chamomile flowers
1/4 cup of ground Oatmeal
1/4 cup of ground Elderflowers
1 teaspoon of honey
1teaspoon Red Clover flower broken apart
1 teaspoon sea salt
First mix all of the dry ingredients together. Then add enough green tea or water to make a mud type paste gently scrub your face and neck with the moist herb mixture. After you have removed the mixture, freshen up with a gentle toner

Lavender vinegar lotion
Steep jointly four ounces of apple cider vinegar, one ounce of lavender flowers, and one ounce of rosemary flowers. Remove the flowers after twenty days. Dilute with eight parts of pure water and use as a cleansing and toning lotion.

Left Over Scrub
I use the plant matter left over from extracts for this one
1 part extract matter such as Witch hazel, Red clover etc.. Use an herb that has skin maintenance properties
½ part sea salt
½ part organic oatmeal
Add a little water so it looks like a thick goop but not pond water and scoop up and handful and scrub away. You can add a drop of essential oil if you want.

Ring Worm
Ringworm is a widespread skin disorder, especially among children, but may occur in people of all ages. Mold-like fungi cause it. It can involve the crotch area, scalp, feet hands, etc...
Some symptoms are reddened skin, itching, and it is ring shaped. As the issue progresses the borders grow as the inside clears.

Topical applications of Black Walnut Hull (Juglans nigra), Pau'D Arco (Tabebuia impetiginosa) Burdock (Arctium lappa) Licorice, Echinacea (Echinacea angustifolia), Oregano these will work well.
Apply topically 3-4 times a day.

You can also take these internally 1-2 times a day.
You can also use essential oils of Thyme (Thymus vulgaris) diluted, Tea tree, neat or Lavender (Lavandula angustifolia).

Impetigo

Impetigo is a skin infection that tends primarily to distress children. Impetigo caused by the bacteria Staphylococcus aureus (also known as staph) affects children of all ages. Impetigo is initiated by the bacteria called group A streptococci (also known as strep) are most common in children ages two to five. The bacteria which cause impetigo are very contagious. They can be spread by a child from one part of his or her body to another by scratching, or contact with a towel, clothing, or stuffed animal. These same methods can pass the bacteria on from one person to another.

Impetigo may be inclined to develop in areas of the skin, which have already been injured through some other mechanism (a cut or scrape, burn, insect bite, or pock from chickenpox).

Internally give a combination of Echinacea (Echinacea purpurea, Echinacea angustifolia), Chickweed, and Astragalus (Astragalus membranaceus) 3 to 4 times per day. Reduce the child's intake of dairy, red meats, and peanut butter, as all have been shown to irritate this illness.

Wash the sores carefully with an infusion made of Calendula (Calendula officinalis) several times per day.
Echinacea tincture can be applied directly to the skin.
The homeopathic remedy Antimonium tartaricum can be used when impetigo is present on the face.
A tincture of the Pansy flower, Viola tricolor, can be taken internally twice daily for a week to speed healing.
Burdock root (Arctium lappa) oil can be directly applied to the skin to help it heal.
Topical washes with Goldenseal (Hydrastis Canadensis), Grapefruit seed extract (which can sting), or Tea Tree (Melaleuca alternifolia) oil are also recommended.

Shampoo Base

This is the base I use for making essential oil shampoos. It makes 2 cups of concentrated shampoo.

Ingredients:
½ cup water
½ cup castile soap
1/2 teaspoon of (extra virgin) olive oil
Method
Mix together all ingredients and place into shampoo bottle. I often mix this using a blender.

Lavender Shampoo
Lavender is a time honored aromatherapy treasure. It soothes an irritated scalp and stimulates the hair follicles. Lavender also aids in relaxation and feelings of well-being.
1/2 cup water
1/2 cup fresh Lavender
2 tablespoons of glycerin
1/2 cup Natural Shampoo Base
Essential Oils- 5 drops of Lavender (Lavandula angustifolia) essential oil
Mix water and lavender together into a heavy bottom pot and bring to a boil.
Let boil gently for at least twenty minutes.
Let cool slightly and add basic shampoo mixture and glycerin slowly to herbal mixture.
Mix well.
Pour shampoo into container and let stand for a few days to allow the mixture to thicken.
Use as you would your regular shampoo.
You can use a simple shampoo base and add any of the following essential oils, Rose, Tea Tree, Lavender, Rosemary, Sandalwood (Santalum album), Palmarosa, Geranium (Pelargonium graveolens) , any scent you desire.

Blonde Highlights Herbal Shampoo Recipe
This shampoo smells like sunshine. Chamomile is well known for its healing properties, is also very effective as a shampoo. It has anti-fungal and antibacterial properties.
1/2 cup Chamomile (Matricaria chamomilla) Flowers
1/2 cup Calendula (Calendula officinalis) Flowers
1-cup tablespoons pure soap flakes
1 1/2 tablespoons glycerin
1 tablespoon Aloe Vera Gel

10 drops Chamomile Essential Oil
Directions:
Boil 1 quart of water- Add flowers. Allow too steep for 3 hours. Strain water into a bowl. Add soap flakes, whisk until incorporated.

Add Aloe and Glycerin. Allow mixture to sit for 1 hour. If mixture is thick enough add essential oil and bottle. If not thick enough, place back in pot reheat add more soap and allow cooling again. Add essential oil when cool.

Brunette Highlights Herbal Shampoo Recipe
This shampoo smells like sunshine. Chamomile is well known for its healing properties, is also very effective as a shampoo. It has anti-fungal and antibacterial properties.
1/2 cup Rosemary Leaf
1/2 cup Nettle Leaf
1-cup tablespoons pure soap flakes
1 1/2 tablespoons glycerin
1 tablespoon Aloe Vera Gel
5 drops Rosemary (Rosmarinus officinalis) or Patchouli (Pogostemon cablin) Essential Oil
Boil 1 quart of water- Add flowers. Allow steeping for 3 hours. Strain water into a bowl. Add soap flakes, whisk until incorporated.
Add Aloe and Glycerin. Allow mixture to sit for 1 hour. If mixture is thick enough add essential oil and bottle. If not thick enough, place back in pot reheat add more soap and allow cooling again. Add essential oil when cool.

Dry Shampoo Recipe
1/2 cup Cornstarch
1-tablespoon fragrant herb powdered, such as rose petals, lavender, sandalwood, and mint.
Blend together well.
Directions- Sprinkle the cornstarch/herb mixture into your hair, let it absorb for a few minutes, brush it out. This is great if you are in a pinch.

Nettle Herbal Hair Rinse
1 cup powdered Nettle
Enough water to make a thin paste, Apply to scalp and hair.
You can add powdered Rosemary also.

Rinse out after 15 minutes.

Brunette Herbal Hair Rinse
Make an infusion
1 part Rosemary
1 part Nettle
1 part Sage
Allow to sit in hair for 15 minutes then rise out.

Insect Remedies
Tick Repellent
4 oz. of water in a spray bottle.
20 drops Eucalyptus EO
20 drops Lemongrass (Cymbopogon citratus) EO
10 drops Clove Bud (Syzygium aromaticum) EO
Spray around ankles, socks, tops of boots and other spaces inviting to ticks.

Mosquito Repellent
4 oz. Tansy (Tanacetum vulgare) tea or other bitter herbs like Barberry (Berberis vulgaris), Yarrow (Achillea millefolium) or Chicory (Cichorium intybus)
10 drops Citronella (Cymbopogon winterianus) EO
10 drops Lemongrass (Cymbopogon citratus) EO
Place in a spray bottle and spray skin and clothing. Assists in repelling gnats, black flies and mosquitoes.

Itch-Away Spray
2 oz. Calendula (Calendula officinalis) Extract
1 oz. Mugwort (Artemisia vulgaris) Extract
1 oz. Cider Vinegar
1 teaspoon Dead Sea Salt
10 drops Eucalyptus (Eucalyptus globulus) EO
10 drops Clove Bud (Syzygium aromaticum) EO
Place in a spray bottle and spray the itchy areas.

7 TEA BLENDS, OXYMELS AND EXTRACTS

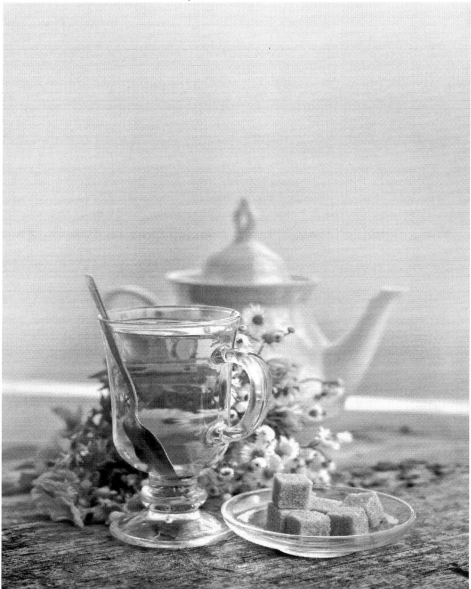

iravgustin /Shutterstock

Women's Teas
Women's Teas for Pregnancy, Labor and Postpartum

YOU ROCK! Mamma Tea and Infusion
2 parts Chamomile flower (Matricaria recutita)
2 parts Hibiscus flower (Hibiscus sabdariffa)
1 part Rose petal (Rosa spp.)
1/8 part Lavender flower (Lavendula officinalis)
1/4 part Rose hips (Rosa canina)
3 parts Lemon balm leaf (Melissa officinalis)
Make this by the gallon. It is rich in nervines, vitamins and minerals. Mom, family and care providers can drink this throughout the day, hot or cold. This is for after birth. It supplies nutrients and vitamins.

Mama Milk
1 part Blessed Thistle (Cnicus benedictus), also known as mothermilk thistle. The herb contains B-complex vitamins, calcium, iron and manganese. Blessed thistle is also a traditional bitter used to aid digestion.
2 parts Nettle (Urtica dioica). Nettles are one of the most widely applicable plants. They strengthen and support the whole body. Throughout Europe, they are used as a spring tonic and general detoxifying remedy. Rich in chlorophyll, iron and calcium, nettles increase breastmilk and energy.
2 parts Red Raspberry leaf (Rubus ideaeus). Red raspberry leaf is rich in calcium, magnesium and iron.
1 part Fennel seed (Foeniculum vulgare). Fennel seed increases the flow of milk.
¼ part Fenugreek (Trigonella foenum-graecum). Fenugreek is an adjunct milk increaser. The chemical components of fenugreek seed include iron, vitamin A, vitamin B1, vitamin C, phosphates, flavonoids, saponins, trigonelline and other alkaloids. This wonderful seed is also high in fiber and protein.
Crush the fenugreek and fennel seeds. Mix ingredients and add 2 teaspoons to a cup of gently simmering water. Simmer for 10 minutes because of the leaf matter that is present.

Mama With a Cold Tea
Sometimes, when mom isn't feeling great, she worries about milk production. This tea can help fortify her milk and treat her cold symptoms.
1 part Rosehips. (Some varieties boast five to 10 times more vitamin C than an orange.) Rosehips are considered depression fighters.

1 part Red Raspberry leaf (Rubus ideaeus)

1 part Red Clover (Trifolium pratense). Red clover contains isoflavins and bioflavonoids. It is considered a gentle blood cleanser.

Prepare as an infusion. Place 2 teaspoons dried plant matter in a cup and add 1 cup of hot water.

Mother Anxiety

1 part Motherwort (Leonurus cardiaca). Motherwort is great for stress and anxiety.

½ part Peppermint (Mentha piperita). Peppermint is great for tension and nervousness.

1 part Nettles (Urtica dioica)

Prepare as an infusion.

Milk Seed Tea

These common seeds are used for milk production all over the world. They are flavorful, too.

1 part Red Raspberry leaf (Rubus ideaeus)

½ part Fennel (Foeniculum vulgare)

½ part Anise (Pimpinella anisum) - increases milk flow

¼ part Caraway (Carum carvi) - increases milk flow

Crush seeds and mix with red raspberry leaf. Prepare as an infusion, because the seeds have a high volatile oil content, and you don't want to be overpowered.

Women's Tea:

1 oz. each of Red Raspberry leaf (Rubus ideaeus), Nettles (Urtica dioica), Melissa (Melissa officinalis), Hibiscus (Hibiscus sabdariffa) flowers, and Spearmint.

1 teaspoon crushed Rose Hips.

1/2teaspoon Stevia if you want it sweeter

This is a bulk blend, so make sure you mix well and store in a clean dry container. Use 2 teaspoon of the blend for each cup of water.

Women's Tea II

1 oz. each Red Raspberry leaf (Rubus ideaeus), Lemongrass (Cymbopogon citratus), Nettles (Urtica dioica) and Melissa (Melissa officinalis).

This is a bulk blend, so make sure you mix well and store in a clean dry container. Use 2 teaspoon of the blend for each cup of water.

Steep for at least 15 minutes

Mother's Milk Tea

1 oz. each Blessed Thistle (Cnicus benedictus)
Fennel seed (Foeniculum vulgare)
Lemongrass (Cymbopogon citratus)
Red Raspberry (Rubus ideaeus) Leaf
Spearmint
Fenugreek seed (Trigonella foenum-graecum)
This is a bulk blend, so make sure you mix well and store in a clean dry container.
Use 2 teaspoon of the blend for each cup of water.
Steep for at least 15 minutes.

Men's Health Teas

Men's Tea

1oz. each of Damiana, Gingko biloba leaf., Kava Kava, Mauria Puama, Oat Straw, Panax Ginseng, Yohimbe Bark, and Peppermint (Mentha piperita) leaf
1 tablespoon crushed Saw Palmetto berries (per two cups of herbs).
1 teaspoon Stevia (per 2 cups of herb)
This is a bulk blend, so make sure you mix well and store in a clean dry container.
Use 2 teaspoon of the blend for each cup of water.
Steep for at least 15 minutes.

Male Strength Tea

1 part Oats (Avena sativa)
1 part Sea Buckthorn (Hippophae rhamnoides)
1 part Nettles (Urtica dioica)
This tea combination promotes overall wellbeing and works well while strength training.

Teas

Immune Boost:

1 oz. each of Alfalfa (Medicago sativa)
Astragalus (Astragalus membranaceus)
Dandelion leaf (Taraxacum officinale)
Milk thistle (Silybum marianum)
Peppermint (Mentha piperita)
Red Clover (Trifolium pratense)
Pau D' Arco (Tabebuia impetiginosa)

Yarrow (Achillea millefolium) flower.

This is a bulk blend, so make sure you mix well and store in a clean dry container.

Use 2 teaspoon of the blend for each cup of water.

Steep for at least 15 minutes.

Sleep Tea

1oz. each of Chamomile, Melissa (Melissa officinalis), Passionflower.

1/4 teaspoon Stevia leaf. (Drink approximately 1 hour before bed).

This is a bulk blend, so make sure you mix well and store in a clean dry container.

Use 2 teaspoon of the blend for each cup of water.

Steep for at least 15 minutes. I myself do not use the stevia, but many people really like it.

Headache Tea

1 oz. each Feverfew, Ginkgo leaf, Ginger, Kava Kava.

1/4 teaspoon Stevia

This is a bulk blend, so make sure you mix well and store in a clean dry container.

Use 2 teaspoon of the blend for each cup of water.

Steep for at least 15 minutes.

Migraine Tea

1 part Feverfew

2 parts Lemon Balm (Melissa officinalis)

1 part Skullcap (Scutellaria lateriflora) (Scutellaria lateriflora)

1 part Passionflower

Make as an infusion. 3-4 cups a day. When you feel a migraine coming on magnesium and B6 supplementation can be helpful. Adding those in our diets can also help prevent migraines.

Throbbing Headache Tea

1 part Rosemary (Rosmarinus officinalis)

2 parts Lemon Balm (Melissa officinalis)

1 part Rose hips

1 part Passionflower

Make as an infusion. 3-4 cups a day.

Urinary Tract Ease

1 oz. each Uva Ursi, Peppermint (Mentha piperita), Slippery Elm.

1/4 teaspoon Stevia
This is a bulk blend, so make sure you mix well and store in a clean dry container.
Use 2 teaspoon of the blend for each cup of water.
Steep for at least 15 minutes.

Willow Bark Pain Relief

2 cups cold water, add 1/2 teaspoon willow bark, soak overnight. In the morning slowly bring to a simmer, turn to low, cover and heat for 20 minutes. Strain. Keeps in fridge 2-3 days. Drink 1/4 cup mixed with your favorite tea 4-5 times per day. *Contains Acetylsalicylic Acid (Aspirin) Use same precautions you would use with aspirin. Do not give to children.

Calming Tea

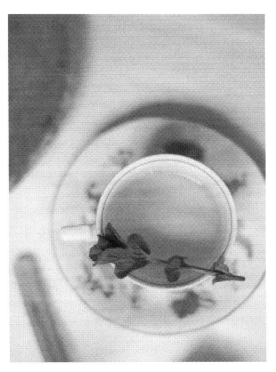

1/2 part Oats (Avena sativa)
1/2 part Catnip (Nepeta cataria)
1/2 part Passion flower (Passiflora incarnata)
1 part Licorice (Glycyrrhiza glabra)
1 part Slippery elm (Ulmus rubra)
2 parts Chamomile (Matricaria chamomilla)
2 parts Spearmint or Peppermint (Mentha piperita)
Make as an infusion, steep for at least 15 minutes.
You can drink this before bed, before a stressful event or something that brings on anxiety.

Sexy Cinnamon Tea

2 parts Cinnamon Bark
1 part Motherwort (Leonurus cardiaca)
½ part Hops (Humulus lupulus)
Make as a decoction and allow too steep for 10-15 minutes. You can drink this when you have a few minutes alone to allow the fire of the cinnamon to build

up onside you. Relax and imagine the fire smoldering inside you. See the fire start at your vagina and imagine it spreading and heating your whole body slowly, branching out.

You can also purchase cinnamon leaves, crush them and leave them in an open container under the bed.

Spring Tonic
Birch leaf tea (Betula Alba) great spring tonic, contributed by 1 teaspoon/cup of water, steep 15 - 20 minutes.

Oxymel Recipes
Cough and Cold Oxymel
Bee Balm (Monarda) and Rosemary (Rosmarinus officinalis), you can do a 50/50 ratio for the herbs.

Fill a small jar about half to three-fourths full of fresh herbs, chopped. Pour honey over the plants and then the vinegar, organic apple cider vinegar. You can use 1/3 honey and the rest vinegar or a 50/50 combination. Stir it all together, it may not easily blend, it will with time. Just stir or shake it every day for about two weeks, then strain well. Bottle into a clean jar. Store, bottle it up and store in a cool place or the refrigerator. Use the highest quality honey you can find. Sustainable and local is really important.

Flu
Garlic, Oregano and Onion, chop the garlic and slice the onion.

Fill a small jar about half to three-fourths full of fresh herbs, chopped. Pour honey over the plants and then the vinegar, organic apple cider vinegar. You can use 1/3 honey and the rest vinegar or a 50/50 combination. Stir it all together, it may not easily blend, it will with time. Just stir or shake it every day for about two weeks, then strain well. Bottle into a clean jar. Store, bottle it up and store in a cool place or the refrigerator. Use the highest quality honey you can find. Sustainable and local is really important.

Sore Throat
Elder Flower (Sambucus nigra), Sage (Salvia officinalis), and Thyme (Thymus vulgaris)

Fill a small jar about half to three-fourths full of fresh herbs, chopped. Pour honey over the plants and then the vinegar, organic apple cider vinegar. You can use 1/3 honey and the rest vinegar or a 50/50 combination. Stir it all together, it may not easily blend, it will with time. Just stir or shake it every day for about two weeks, then strain well. Bottle into a clean jar. Store, bottle it up and store in a cool place or the refrigerator. Use the highest quality honey you can find. Sustainable and local is really important.

Pregnancy Oxymel

Red Raspberry (Rubus ideaeus), Alfalfa (Medicago sativa) and Nettles (Urtica dioica).

Fill a small jar about half to three-fourths full of fresh herbs, chopped. Pour honey over the plants and then the vinegar, organic apple cider vinegar.

You can use 1/3 honey and the rest vinegar or a 50/50 combination. Stir it all together, it may not easily blend, it will with time. Just stir or shake it every day for about two weeks, then strain well. Bottle into a clean jar. Store, bottle it up and store in a cool place or the refrigerator. Use the highest quality honey you can find. Sustainable and local is really important.

Morning Sickness Oxymel

Peppermint (Mentha piperita) and Spearmint (also good for upset stomachs). Ginger Root

Fill a small jar about half to three-fourths full of fresh herbs, chopped. Pour honey over the plants and then the vinegar, organic apple cider vinegar.

You can use 1/3 honey and the rest vinegar or a 50/50 combination. Stir it all together, it may not easily blend, it will with time. Just stir or shake it every day for about two weeks, then strain well. Bottle into a clean jar. Store, bottle it up and store in a cool place or the refrigerator. Use the highest quality honey you can find. Sustainable and local is really important.

Ginger, Garlic & Onion Oxymel

In a jar fill with sliced onions, white or yellow, packed in well. Sweet onions do not seem to work as well. Add to it grated ginger, and sliced garlic to fill in the cracks. Make sure you have plenty of room left to cover all with honey. Allow this too steep for 2 weeks and strain and add almost an equal amount of vinegar. You can also add some fresh lemon or orange peel. This can also be made as a glycerite. This is good for coughs, sore throats and overall health and wellbeing.

Other Herbs that are great in Oxymels.

Bee Balm (Monarda): sore throat, antibacterial, helpful for thick congested coughs, or fever.

Peppermint, Spearmint: These herbs are known for easing digestive complaints, upset stomach and helpful for nausea.

Elder flowers and buds: specific for sore throats, and immune stimulating.

Oregano: Oregano is coveted in so many societies because it is antibacterial, antiviral, and beneficial for upper respiratory infections and fungal issues.

Rosemary: Helpful for issues affecting energy levels and circulation issues, this can be supportive for digestion and the nervous system and memory. Limit use when pregnant, avoid daily or medicinal use, that being said in many countries women eat Rosemary every day, fresh, in salads and savory dishes.

Raspberry Leaves: Overall Raspberry leaves are considered one of the best women's tonic herbs, mildly astringent, and full of nutrients. Helpful for menstrual issues, PMS, and menopause issues.

Sage: is a helpful antifungal, antibacterial, antiviral herb. *Contraindications*: not for breastfeeding, it inhibits milk flow, not use by pregnant or nursing women.

Thyme: often used for upper respiratory infections, bronchitis, coughs antiviral and antibacterial.

Ginger: Shredded ginger, is great for nausea and digestion in an oxymel.

Echinacea: Respiratory tract infections, use the fresh root, for optimal results.

Extract Blend Recipes

You can find tincture and extract recipes all over and in most herbal books. I am just sharing a few of mine I really like. I could fill hundreds of pages with just extract blends.

Glycerite Stress Extract

2 parts Passionflower (Passiflora incarnata)
1 part Chamomile (Matricaria recutita)
1 part Lemon Balm (Melissa officinalis)

½ part Catnip (Nepeta cataria) and Lavender (Lavandula angustifolia)
Make as a glycerite. Use 1 teaspoon 3-4 times a day.

Women's Health Glycerite Extract
1 oz. each Red Raspberry (Rubus ideaeus) leaf, Lemongrass (Cymbopogon citratus), Nettles (Urtica dioica) and Melissa (Melissa officinalis). Make as a glycerite and use 1 teaspoon 3-4 times a day. You can also make as an oxymel.

Men's Health Glycerite Extract
1 part Dandelion Leaf-fresh (Taraxacum officinale)
1 part Lemon Balm (Melissa officinalis)-fresh
1 part Ginger Root- fresh
Make as a glycerite and use 1 teaspoon 3-4 times a day.
You can also make as an oxymel.
This is great for men's overall health.

Vitamin and Mineral Glycerite Extract
2 parts Rose Hips
2 parts Nettle (Urtica dioica)
2 parts Dandelion Leaf (Taraxacum officinale)
½ part Cinnamon
Make as a glycerite. I would personally make in at least a quart size. Use enough herb to almost fill the jar, leave an inch for expansion, cover with vegetable glycerin and allow too steep for 3-6 weeks. Strain and use 2 tablespoons a day. You could also make this as an oxymel or extract.
This is beneficial for overall health and wellbeing.

Acne Extract
1 part Dandelion Root (Taraxacum officinale)
1 part Nettles (Urtica dioica)
1 part Echinacea Root (Echinacea angustifolia)
20-30 drops 3 times a day. Make as an extract. I have used this blend with many a teenager, internally and topically.

Anxiety Blend
2 parts Borage (Borago officinalis)
2 parts St. John's Wort flower (Hypericum perforatum)
1 part Hawthorn berry (Crataegus oxyacantha & C. monogyna)

1 part Milky Oats (Avena Sativa)
Make as an extract. 30 drops, 2-3 times a day.

Anxiety Blend II
1 part Motherwort (Leonurus cardiaca)
1 part Linden (Tilia europea)
1 part Skullcap (Scutellaria lateriflora herb)
Make as an extract. 30 drops, 2-3 times a day.

Gassy Guts Extract
1 part Ceylon Cinnamon bark (Cinnamomun aromaticum)
1 part Nutmeg seed (Myristica fragrans)
1/2 part Fennel
Make as an extract use 20-30 drops before or after eating to help prevent gas.

Iron Extract
1 part Alfalfa (Medicago sativa)
1 part Dandelion (Taraxacum officinale)
1 part Nettle (Urtica dioica)
1 part Yellow Dock (Rumex crispus)
Make as an extract, 30-40 drops 3 times a day
This contains iron rich herbs.

Intestinal Defense
2 parts Black Walnut (Juglans nigra)
1 part Sweet Wormwood (Artemisia annua)
1 part Quassia wood (Quassia amara)
½ part Clove flower bud (Syzgium aromaticum)
2 parts Cardamom seed w/pod (Elettaria cardamomum)
2 parts Ginger rhizome, fresh (Zingiber officinale)
Make as an extract. 1-2 teaspoons 2-3 times a day for a week.

Joint Care Blend
1 part Devil's Claw root (Harpagophytum procumbens)
1 part Ginger root (Zingiber officinale)
1 part Turmeric root (Curcuma longa)
1 part Yucca root (Yucca glauca)
½ part Oats (Avena Sativa)

Make as an extract. 30 drops 3 times a day.
This is wonderful in my opinion for deep joint pain, and lower back pain.

Overall Adrenal Support Extract
2 parts Eleuthero root (Eleutherococcus senticosus)
2 parts Milky Oats (Avena sativa)
1 part Nettles (Urtica dioica)
1 part Licorice root (Glycyrrhiza glabra)
1 part Sarsaparilla root (Smilax (ornata) regelii)
1/2 part Prickly Ash bark (Zanthoxylum clava-herculis)
30 drops 3 times a day. Make as an extract
Offers overall adrenal support.

Pain Formula Extract
2 parts Turmeric (Curcuma longa)
1 part Skullcap leaf & flower (Scutellaria lateriflora)
1 part Cramp bark (Viburnum opulus)
1 part Black Cohosh root (Cimicifuga racemosa)
½ part Yarrow (Achillea millefolium)
This us nice for deep pain. I have used it topically and internally.

Sleepytime Extract Blend
1 part Oats (Avena sativa)
1 part Chamomile flower (Matricaria recutita)
1 part Hops (Humulus lupulus)
1 part Skullcap leaf & flower (Scutellaria lateriflora)
1 part Rose hips (Rosa sp.)
Make as an extract. 40 drops before bed.

7 Around the Home

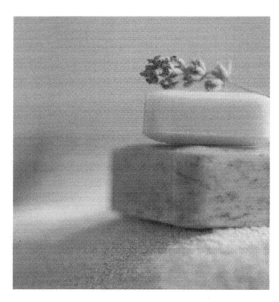

Household Cleaners
Tub scrub
1 cup borax
10 drops tea tree
Use like you would a traditional abrasive tub cleaner. Make sure it will not scratch fiberglass, or stain.

Bathroom Wipes
Paper towels (1/2 regular roll)
1 cup castile soap
1 tablespoon Pine (Pinus sylvestris) essential oil
1 tablespoon Lemon essential oil.
2 cups water

Mix well.
Unwrap the paper towels and stack them in a tub container with a well-fitting lid. Fold the towels in the containers and pour the mixture over the towels. Use them as you would wipes. I like to use cut flannel clothes instead of paper towels and I can wash and reuse them.

Heavy Duty Bathroom Cleaner:
3/4 c. baking soda
¼ cup lemon juice
3 tablespoons salt
3 tablespoons liquid dishwashing soap, or castile soap
1/2 cup vinegar

10 drops Tea Tree (Melaleuca alternifolia) essential oil.

10 drops Lavender (Lavandula angustifolia) essential oil.

In a medium bowl, mix together and make a paste. Use scrubby sponge, or brush to apply to the side of the tub, shower walls, and sinks. (Be sure to test a small out of site area to make sure paste does not scratch tub surface; if that does occur, you can remove salt from the mixture). Rinse well, and use a wet towel to remove.

Toilet Bowl Cleaner

Borax

Lemon juice

Mix the lemon juice and borax salts to make a paste about the consistency of toothpaste or a really thick cold cream. Flush toilet to wet sides. Rub paste on toilet bowl ring. Let sit for 2 hours and then scrub thoroughly. You can add a few drops of Peppermint (Mentha piperita), lemon or Rosemary (Rosmarinus officinalis) essential oils if you would like.

Window Cleaner

1/4 cup vinegar

10 drops Tea tree, Lavender, Rosemary (Rosmarinus officinalis) or Peppermint (Mentha piperita)

1 quart water

Add to a spray bottle and use just like commercial window cleaner.

Window Wipes

Roll Paper Towels (1/2 regular roll)

1 cup homemade glass cleaner- above

1 1/2 cups water

10 drops Tea Tree (Melaleuca alternifolia) or Rosemary (Rosmarinus officinalis) essential oil.

Unwrap the paper towels and stack them in a tub container with a well-fitting lid. Fold the towels in the containers and pour the mixture over the towels. Use them as you would window wipes.

Stainless Steel Sink Cleaner

1 cup salt

1 cup Baking Soda

Sprinkle onto a cloth or sponge and clean the area.

Drain Cleaner

1/2 cup baking soda

1/2 cup white vinegar

1 teaspoon tea tree

Boiling water

Pour the baking soda into the drain, and add the teaspoon tea tree. Pour over the vinegar. The drain will foam, allow it to sit for a half an hour. After the drain sits for a half an hour flush the drain with a kettle of boing water.

Be careful. Do not burn yourself.

Sick wash

I use this for toilet seats, doorknobs, etc. when everyone is sick. It is great as an overall cleaning solution when we have flues and colds.

1/4 cup water

1/8 cup vodka

1 teaspoon Tea Tree (Melaleuca alternifolia) EO

1 teaspoon Lavender (Lavandula angustifolia), Rosemary (Rosmarinus officinalis) or Peppermint (Mentha piperita)

You can put this in a large spray bottle.

Furniture Cleaner and Polish

3 cups olive oil

1 cup vinegar or lemon juice

Mix together until well blended. Use a clean, soft cloth to apply to the furniture. Apply to a test area before using on any surfaces.

Brass Cleaner

Lemon juice

Baking soda

Make a paste about the consistency of toothpaste. Rub onto brass with a soft cloth. Rinse with water and dry.

Brass Cleaner

Lemon juice

Cream of tartar

Make a paste about the consistency of toothpaste. Apply to surface, leave on for 5 minutes. Wash with warm water. Dry with a soft cloth.

Carpet Cleaner
2 cups baking soda
1/2 teaspoon essential oil your choice.
Shake well. Allow to sit for a 1/2 hour, then sprinkle, allow to dry and vacuum. You can use Cedarwood, Lavender, Eucalyptus or Sweet Orange EO to repel fleas.

No-Wax Linoleum Cleaner
1 tablespoon white vinegar
1 gallon warm water
20 drops Lemon/Tea Tree (Melaleuca alternifolia) or Rosemary (Rosmarinus officinalis) essential oil.
Mix together in a bucket.
Mop as you normally would.

Super Cleaning Spray
1/2 cup white vinegar
2 teaspoons Borax
1/4 cup liquid soap
40 ounces hot water
20-30 drops Lavender (Lavandula angustifolia) essential oil
Mix all together and put in a spray bottle for use.
I use this on really grimy woodwork, and doors.

Shoe Freshener
I use on my stinky Danskos. When you are attending births and getting all kinds of matter on your shoes, and it is nice to be able to have them clean and smelling fresh.
5 drops Lavender (Lavandula angustifolia) EO
5 drops tea tree
1 tablespoon baking powder
1/8 cup water.
Put in spray bottle, mix well. Gentle mist and allow to dry overnight.
I have also used this on construction boots so with that type of stank I use a q-tip and get the leather creases, insoles, etc... Make sure you patch test to make sure that the cleaner will not ruin your shoes.

Laundry Soap
1 large box borax
1 small box baking soda
2 boxes Ivory soap flakes
5 teaspoons Lavender and Tea Tree (Melaleuca alternifolia) essential oil, you decide the combination. This is what I used on cloth diapers. I used this detergent or variations of it for years and I only stopped when I moved to Europe and couldn't find all of the ingredients.
Mix all together. Cover and let sit for 48 hours before using. I would use a 1/8 cup a load or even less, depending on the load.

Baby Wipes
Paper towels (1/2 regular roll) I use wash clothes that it quickly dab in my prepared solution.
2 1/4 cups water
1 tablespoons liquid castile soap
2 teaspoons olive oil or apricot kernel oil (I used infused Calendula (Calendula officinalis) oil)
10 drops Lavender (Lavandula angustifolia) or German Chamomile.

Face/Hand Wipes
Paper towels (1/2 regular roll)
2 tablespoons liquid castile soap
2 cups water
Place this in a sealable container with the paper towels for use later, or use with cotton flannel clothes.

Diffuser Blends- Any of the oil blends can be used as a diffuser blends.

Potpourri
Potpourri is essentially using herbs to introduce smell into the environment in a steady manner that is not overpowering. It uses dried herbs generally in a pretty bowl or basic. Some people add fragrance oils to blend, I think this smells too artificial, but at times I have added a few drops of essential oil to freshen the blend.

Exotic Scents can be made by using:
Sandalwood

Rose Petals
Jasmine Flowers
Orange Flowers
Cinnamon
Clove
Anise
Coriander
Cardamom

Outdoorsy Scent Potpourri
Pine Needles
Pine Bark
Cedar Shavings
Chamomile
Meadowsweet
Hay
Rosemary
Bay
Eucalyptus Leaf
Red Sandalwood chips

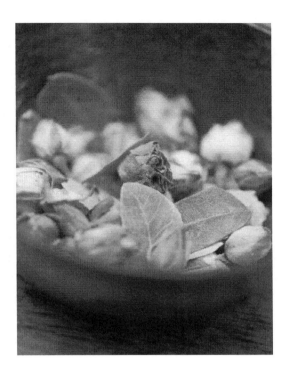

Citrus Potpourri
Lemon Balm
Lemon Verbena
Orange Peel
Lemon Peel
Kumquats dried
Lemon Grass

Refreshing Potpourri
Peppermint
Spearmint
Wintergreen
Birch bark and leaf
Mix your desired herbs in a bowl, sprinkle with a drop or two of complimentary essential oil. Place in a decorative container.

Sexy Potpourri
1 part Rose petals
1 part Jasmine flower
½ part Cedar shavings

Sachets
A sachet is a small fabric bag filled with fragrant herbs. Most are bags, 4 inches by 4 inches and tied off with ribbon. You fill the bag with the fragrant dried herbs and place the bag in linen closets, dressers, and closets.

Sachets have a recorder history that spans as far back as the Han Dynasty in China. Sachets have been used to scent garments and people, ward off evil spirits and protects items from bugs, worms and other pests one could find in a linen closet.

Southern Woods Sachet
1 cup Woodruff
1/2 cup Agrimony
3/4 cup Southernwood
6 crumbled Bay Leaves
5 teaspoons Rosemary leaves
1 tablespoon Orris Root
Mix well and add to a sachet. Tie and place in closets, linen cupboards, and drawers.

Romantic Dreams Sachet
1 cup Lavender flowers
1 cup Rose Petals
2 teaspoons Cedar shavings
1/2 cup Lemon Verbena (Aloysia citriodora)
1 tablespoon Rosemary leaf
2 teaspoons crushed Cinnamon
1 tablespoon Orris Root
Mix well and add to a sachet. Tie and place in closets, linen cupboards, and drawers.

Dream Sachet
1 cup Hops (Humulus lupulus)
1/2 cup Woodruff

1/2 cup Chamomile flower
Place under pillow, mattress or in your room to promote sleep.

Dream Deeply
1 cup Hops (Humulus lupulus)
1/2 cup Mugwort (Artemisia vulgaris)
1/2 cup Lavender flower
1/4 cup Agrimony
Place under pillow, mattress or in your room to promote deep sleep.

Fresh and Clean Sachet
1 cup Lavender Flower
1 cup Spearmint Leaf
Mix well and add to a sachet. Tie and place under pillow, beside the bed on a bedside table, or under the bed.

Lemon Fresh Sachets
1 cup Lemon Verbena (Aloysia citriodora)
1/2 cup Spearmint Leaf
1/2 cup Orange peel
Mix well and add to a sachet. Tie and place in closets, linen cupboards, and drawers

Moth Bag Sachet
1 part Wormwood
1 part Southernwood
1 part Lavender
1 part Pennyroyal
1 part Tansy
Mix well and add to a sachet. Tie and place in closets, linen cupboards, and drawers, or storage closet.

Moth Bag II
1 part Lemon Verbena (Aloysia citriodora)
1 part Rosemary
1 part Rue
1 part Sage
1 part Wormwood

Mix well and add to a sachet. Tie and place in closets, linen cupboards, and drawers. If you have a wool suit you can tie the sachet around the coat hanger hook and put a small sachets in the pockets to ward off critters. Wool is a favorite of moths.

Hanging Herbal Blends
These can have two purposes, decorative or useful.
Useful hangings- These are hangings that can be in the kitchen for use in food preparation.
5 sprigs about 10 inches long Rosemary
5- 8 inch long stems of Oregano
5 8 inch stems Sage
Hang and allow to dry. Upon them completely drying, place in jars. Store properly and use as needed. You can also just use straight off the hangings.

Beautiful Day Hanging Herbs
5 springs Lavender
5 sprigs Sweet Annie
5 sprigs Statice- Purple or White
2 dried Hydrangea
Form and wrap into a bouquet.
You can also use Calendula (Calendula officinalis), Queen Anne's lace, and other fragrant or structurally interesting herbs.

Pinks- Hanging Herbs
Use an assortment of the following that have been dried, Strawflowers, Nigella, Statice, Rosemary, Sage, and Lavender.
Make a bouquet to hang or make a wreath, or swag.

Linens
Linen Spray
My all-time favorite way to refresh linens is to hang them in the sun, but this does not always work if you have unexpected company, rainy weather or winter climates. The sun though does act as a natural disinfectant, and nothing smells better in my mind than fresh warm linens off the line.

Linen sprays have a long tradition of use. They have been used to refresh linens, musty guest rooms and closets. Here are the basic instructions for a linen spray and then suggestions for recipes. Of course you can formulate your own.

In a large measuring cup or glass bowl pour the following:
3 oz. Alcohol Isopropyl, Higher proof Vodka or Clear Witch Hazel.
25-40 drops of essential oil
1 1/2 cups distilled water
Mix well, and add to a spray bottle. Mist your linens to keep them smelling fresh. This is a basic recipe for a linen spray. Certain essential oils work well with certain kinds of linen.
These are my suggestions.

Duvet Linen Spray

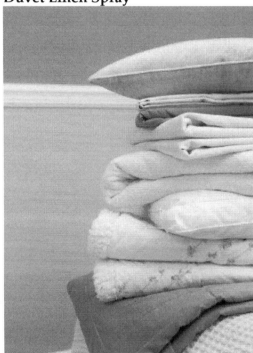

3 oz. Alcohol Isopropyl, Higher proof Vodka or Clear Witch Hazel.
15 drops Sweet Orange (Citrus sinensis) essential oil
20 drops Lavender essential oil
1 1/2 cups distilled water
Mist your duvet, wait 30 minutes and place the cover on and fluff.

Sunshine Towels

3 oz. Alcohol Isopropyl, Higher proof Vodka or Clear Witch Hazel.
15 drops Lemon essential oil
15 drops Spearmint essential oil
1 1/2 cups distilled water
Mist your towels and fold 30 minutes later.

Cloth Diaper Clean!

3 oz. Alcohol Isopropyl, Higher proof Vodka or Clear Witch Hazel.
15 drops Lavender essential oil
20 drops Peppermint (Mentha piperita) essential oil
1 1/2 cups distilled water
When the diapers have been washed and dried, before folding, mist lightly. After 30 minutes fold the diapers and they are ready for use. Sometimes the

bacteria trapped in even the best washed diapers leaves a residual smell. This can help with that.

Sleepytime Bed Linen
3 oz. Alcohol Isopropyl, Higher proof Vodka or Clear Witch Hazel.
15 drops Lemon balm (Melissa officinalis) essential oil
15 drops Lavender (Lavandula angustifolia) essential oil
10 drops Chamomile (Matricaria chamomilla)
1 1/2 cups distilled water
When replacing the sheets, while the sheets are off, mist your mattress lightly and replace your sheets.

Curtain Spray
Refresh your curtains by giving them a little spritz after laundering, or when they need a little revitalizing.
3 oz. Alcohol Isopropyl, Higher proof Vodka or Clear Witch Hazel.
15 drops Peppermint (Mentha piperita) essential oil
15 drops Lemon essential oil
1 1/2 cups distilled water
Spritz your curtains after laundering and rehanging.

9 RESOURCES

Herbal Schools
Heart of Herbs Herbal School
501 Lindsey St.
Reidsville, NC 27320
866-303-4372
www.heartofherbs.com
This school is directed by the books
author- Demetria Clark

Sage Mountain- Rosemary Gladstar
Barre, VT
www.sagemountain.com

Wise Woman Center and Susun
Weed
Woodstock, NY
www.susunweed.com

David Winston's Center for Herbal
Studies
www.herbalstudies.org

East West School of Herbology
www.planetherbs.com

Herbal Suppliers
Mountain Rose Herbs
www.mountainroseherbs.com
Frontier Co-op
www.frontiercoop.com

Starwest Botanicals
www.Starwest-Botanicals.com

Bulk Herb Store
www.bulkherbstore.com

Stony Mountain Botanicals
www.wildroots.com

Fresh Herbs and Seeds

Horizon Herbs
www.horizonherbs.com

Richters
www.richters.com

Essential Oils
Mountain Rose Herbs
www.mountainroseherbs.com

Nature's Gift
www.naturesgift.com

The Essential Oil Company
www.essentialoil.com

Aura Cacia
www.auracacia.com

Swiss Aromatics
originalswissaromatics.com

SunRose Aromatics
www.sunrosearomatics.com

Lab of Flowers
www.laboffowers.com

Carrier Oils
Mountain Rose Herbs
www.mountainroseherbs.com

Frontier Co-op
www.frontiercoop.com

Bulk Apothecary
www.bulkapothecary.com

Essential Wholesale
www.essentialwholesale.com

From Nature with Love
www.fromnaturewithlove.com/

Herbs and Herb Plants

Adaptations

808-328-9044

Permaculture-grown tropical plants, including ginger, gotu kola, kava, and passionflower.

Frontier Natural Products Co-op

www.frontiercoop.com

Garden Medicinals

www.gardenmedicinals.com

Horizon Herbs

www.horizonherbs.com

Medicinal Herb Plants

www.medicinalherbplants.com

Mountain Rose Herbs

www.mountainroseherbs.com

Nature's Cathedral

www.naturescathedral.com

Echinacea, goldenseal, and other cultivated herbs.

Pacific Botanicals

www.pacificbotanicals.com

High-quality organic and wildcrafted herbs. Will deliver fresh plants.

Richters Herbs

www.richters.com

Southern Virginia Herbals - Certified Organic

1107 Wooding Trail

Halifax, VA 24558

Tel: (804) 476-1339

Fax: (804) 476-4413

www.gardenmedicinals.com/pages/va_sources.html

Organic herbs from the East and Southeast.

Chinese Herbs

Spring Wind Herbs
www.springwind.com

Starwest Botanicals

www.starwest-botanicals.com

Herb Seeds

Abundant Life Seeds

www.abundantlifeseeds.com

Johnny's Selected Seeds

www.johnnyseeds.com

Bountiful Gardens

www.bountifulgardens.org

Seed Savers Exchange

www.seedsavers.org

Fedco Seeds

www.fedcoseeds.com

Seeds From Italy

www.growitalian.com

Harris Seeds

www.harrisseeds.com

Seeds of Change

www.seedsofchange.com

High Mowing Organic Seeds

www.highmowingseeds.com

Territorial Seed Company

www.territorialseed.com

Bottles and Containers

Acme Vial & Glass Company, Inc.

www.acmevial.com

Berlin Packaging

www.berlinpackaging.com

BASCO

www.bascousa.com

Cape Bottle Company

www.netbottle.com

Cleveland Bottle & Supply Co.

www.clevelandbottle.com

E. D. Luce Packaging

www.essentialsupplies.com

General Bottle Supply

www.bottlesetc.com

Industrial Container and Supply Company

www.industrialcontainer.com

Mid-Continent AgriMarketing, Inc.

800-547-1392

Also supplies beeswax, dyes, jars, molds, and scents.

Packaging West, Inc.

www.tricorbraun.com

SKS Bottle & Packaging, Inc.

www.sks-bottle.com

Also supplies droppers, jars, salves, and tins.

Sunburst Bottle Company

www.sunburstbottle.com

Other Supplies and Ingredients

Bramble Berry Soap Making Supplies

www.brambleberry.com

Columbus Foods

www.soaperschoice.com

From Nature with Love

www.fromnaturewithlove.com

Liberty Natural Products, Inc.

www.libertynatural.com

Rainbow Meadow, Inc.

www.rainbowmeadow.com

Western Plastics Corp.

www.uscontainer.com

Bean Tree Soaps

www.beantreesoap.com

Motherlove Herbal Company

www.motherlove.com

Botanical Earth

www.botanicalearth.com

Mountain Rose Herbs

www.mountainroseherbs.com

Dreamseeds Organics

http://hyenacart.com/dreamseeds

Great Cape Herbs

www.greatcape.com

San Francisco Herb Co.

www.sfherb.com

Stony Mountain Botanicals

www.wildroots.com

Maine Coast Herbals

www.maineherbs.com

WiseWays Herbals

www.wiseways.com

Vinegar

Bragg Live Foods

www.bragg.com

Sonoma Vinegar Works

www.sonomavinegarworks.com

American Herb Association

www.ahaherb.com

American Herbalists Guild

www.americanherbalistguild.com

Herb Research Foundation

www.herbs.org

National Association for Holistic Aromatherapy

www.naha.org

United Plant Savers

www.unitedplantsavers.org

Associations and Schools

Herb Associations

Books

For more information about making herbal and aromatherapy remedies:

Arnould-Taylor, W. E. A Textbook of Holistic Aromatherapy: The Use of Essential Oils Treatments. Philadelphia, PA: Trans-Atlantic Publications, 1992.

Cech, R. Making Plant Medicine. Williams, OR: Horizon Herbs, 2000.

Close, B. Aromatherapy: The A–Z Guide to Healing with Essential Oils. New York: Dell, 1997.

Clark, Demetria. 475 Herbal and Aromatherapy Recipes, Heart of Herbs School, NC 2013.

Dodt, C., and D. Balmuth. Essential Oils Book: Creating Personal Blends for Mind and Body. North Adams, MA: Storey Publishing, 1996.

Fischer-Rizzi, S. Complete Aromatherapy Handbook: Essential Oils for Radiant Health. New York: Sterling, 1991.

Gattefosse, R., and R. Tisserand. Gattefosse's Aromatherapy: The First Book on Aromatherapy. London: Random House, 2004.

Gladstar, R. Rosemary Gladstar's Herbal Recipes for Vibrant Health: 175 Teas, Tonics, Oils, Salves, Tinctures, and Other Natural Remedies for the Entire Family. North Adams, MA: Storey Publishing, 2008.

Grace, U. Aromatherapy for Practitioners. London: C. W. Daniel, 2009.

Green, J. Herbal Medicine Maker's Handbook: A Home Manual. Freedom, CA: Crossing Press, 2000.

Grieve, M. Modern Herbal (Volume 1, A–H) and A Modern Herbal (Volume 2, H–Z). Whitefish, MT: Kessinger, 2006.

Hoffman, D. Herbal Handbook: A User's Guide to Medical Herbalism. Rochester, VT: Healing Arts Press, 1998.

Mabey, R., and M. McIntyre. New Age Herbalist: How to Use Herbs for Healing, Nutrition, Body Care, and Relaxation. New York: Fireside, 1988.

Schnaubelt, K. Advanced Aromatherapy. Rochester, VT: Healing Arts Press, 1995.

Schnaubelt, K. Medical Aromatherapy. Berkeley, CA: Frog Ltd., 1999.

Tisserand, M. Aromatherapy for Women: A Practical Guide to Essential Oils for Health and Beauty. Rochester, VT: Healing Arts Press, 1988.

Tisserand, R. Aromatherapy. London: C. W. Daniel, 2004.

Tisserand, R., and T. Balacs. Essential Oil Safety. London: Churchill Livingstone, 1995.

Valnet, J., and R. Tisserand. Practice of Aromatherapy: A Classic Compendium of Plant Medicines and Their Healing Properties. Rochester, VT: Healing Arts Press, 1982.

For more information about growing your own herbs:

Brennan, G. Little Herb Gardens: Simple Secrets for Glorious Gardens Indoors and Out. San Francisco: Chronicle Books, 2004.

Cech, R. Growing At-Risk Medicinal Herbs, Cultivation, Conservation, and Ecology. Williams, OR: Horizon Herbs, 2002.

De La Tour, S. Herbalist's Garden: A Guided Tour of 10 Exceptional Herb Gardens, The People Who Grow Them and the Plants That Inspire Them. North Adams, MA: Storey Publishing, 2001.

Hirsch, D. Moosewood Restaurant Kitchen Garden. Berkeley, CA: Ten Speed Press, 2005.

Kavasch, E. B. Medicine Wheel Garden: Creating Sacred Space for Healing, Celebration, and Tranquility. New York: Bantam, 2002.

McIntyre, A. Good Health Garden: Growing and Using Healing Foods. New York: Reader's Digest, 1998.

Smith, M. Your Backyard Herb Garden: A Gardener's Guide to Growing over 50 Herbs Plus How to Use Them in Cooking, Crafts, Companion Planting, and More. Emmaus, PA: Rodale, 1999.

Sombke, L. Beautiful Easy Herbs: How to Get the Most from Herbs—In Your Garden and in Your Home. Emmaus, PA: Rodale, 2000.

Sturdivant, L., and T. Blakley. The Bootstrap Guide to Medicinal Herbsvin the Garden, Field, and Marketplace. Friday Harbor, WA: San Juan Naturals, 1998.

ABOUT THE AUTHOR

Demetria Clark lives in NC with her husband, sons, two cats, a dog and frog. She spends her time working at Heart of Herbs Herbal School www.heartofherbs.com and Birth Arts International, www.birtharts.com She is also the author of Herbal Healing for Children. She believes in love and family first in all things.

INDEX

Absolute, 13

Acne Extract, 159

Acne Toner, 138

Acne, Blemish Remover Formula, 138

Acute Pain- For Joint Pain, 50

Ajowan, 18

Almond, Bitter, 18

Angelica Root, 21

Antique Queen of Hungary Water. *Queen of Hungary Water*

Anxiety Blend, 160

Anxiety Blend II, 160

Arnica, 18

Arnica Calendula Liniment, 130

Arnica Calendula Oil, 131

Arnica Liniment, 129

Arnica Liniment II, 130

Arnica SJW Oil, 130

Arthritis Blend, 51

Arthritis Blend II, 52

Arthritis Massage Oil, 51

Arthritis Oils, 51

Athlete's Foot Sea Salt Soak, 92

Athletes Foot Vinegar Liniment, 133

Baby Wipes. *Household Cleaners*

Back Ache Massage Oil, 52

Balancing Oil. Infused Oil Blends

BATH SALTS, 73

Bath Salts- Basic Base Recipe. *BATH SALTS*

Bathroom Wipes. *Household Cleaners*

Beautiful Day Hanging Herbs, 171

Bergamot, 21

Bhringaraj Oil. *Infused Oil Blends*

Birch, Sweet, 18

Bitter Orange, 21

Black Walnut Salve. *Skin Issue Salves*

Blonde Highlights Herbal Shampoo Recipe, 144

Body Sprays, 93

Boldo Leaf, 19

Brahmi Oil. *Infused Oil Blends*

Brass Cleaner. *Household Cleaners, Household Cleaners*

Brewing Guide, 26

Broom, Spanish, 19

Brunette Highlights Herbal Shampoo Recipe, 145

Bubble Bath, 88

BUYING HERBS, 23

Cabbage Poultice. *Poultice*

Calamus, 19

Calendula St. John's Wort Oil, 131

Calendula St. St. John's Wort Oil, 131

Callous Balm, 125

Calming Tea, 155

Calming Tea Bath, 89

Camphor Wowzer Balm, 124

Camphor, Brown, 19

Carpet cleaner. *Household Cleaners*

Carrier Oils, 22, 46

Cayenne Muscle Salve, 123

Circulation Massage Oil, 53

Circulation Oil 2, 53

Citrus Massage Oil, 68

Citrus Potpourri. *Potpourri*

Cleansing and Detox Mud Bath. *Bubble Bath*

Cleansing Breath Massage Oil, 69

Closeness Oil. *Infused Oil Blends*

Cloth Diaper Clean!, 172

Colds and Flu, 54

Commonly Infused Herbs. *Infused Oils*

Compress, 33

Congestion Balm, 126

Coping with New Responsibilities- Great for the overwhelmed Mom or Dad., 94

Cottonwood Liniment, 131

Cough and Cold Oxymel, 155

Cracked Skin Salve. *Skin Issue Salves*

Cradle Cap, 63

Cradle Cap blend, 127

Creams. *See*

Crockpot method or electric roaster method. *Infused Oils*

Cucumber Astringent, 139

Cumin, 21

Curtain Spray, 173

Dead Sea Salts. *BATH SALTS*

Decoctions, 26

DeStress and Rest Bath Oil, 86

Dill Seed, 21

Distillation, 14

Do It Yourself Scrub, 141

Double boiler method. *Infused Oils*

Drain Cleaner. *Household Cleaners*

Dream Deeply. *Sachets*

Dream Sachet. *Sachets*

DreamTouch Massage Oil. *Medicinal Oils with Essential Oil*

Dry Shampoo Recipe, 145

Dry Skin. *Infused Oil Blends*

Duvet Linen Spray, 172

Easy Lotion Bar, 67

Eczema Oil. *Infused Oil Blends*

Electuary, 29

Energizing Bath Salts. *BATH SALTS*

Energizing Sea Salt Scrub, 82

Energy Booster, 93

Enfleurage. *Extraction Methods of Essential Oils*

Enhancing Self-Love, 94

Enlightened Bath Oil, 84

Epsom. *BATH SALTS*

Essential Oil Blends for Emotional Issues, 95

Essential Oil Quality, 15

Essential Oil Storage, 17

Essential Oil, Extraction, 13

Exotic Nights, 70

Exotic Salts. *BATH SALTS*

Expression. *Extraction Methods of Essential Oils*

Extra Rich Lotion Bar, 67

Extract Blend Recipes, 158

Extraction Methods of Essential Oils, 13

Extracts, 27

Face/Hand Wipes. *Household Cleaners*

Floral Tea Bath, 90

Flu, 156

Fomentation. *Poultice*

For Him, 70

Fragrant Bath Salts. *Bath Salts*

Fresh and Clean Sachet. *Sachets*

Fungal Infection Liniment, 133

Furniture Cleaner and Polish. *Household Cleaners*

Garlic, 19

Gentle Life Sea Salt Scrub, 82

Ginger Liniment, 131

Ginger, Garlic & Onion Oxymel, 157

Glycerin Herbal Extracts, 29

Glycerite Stress Extract, 158

Goddess Face Scrub, 141

Goldenseal Calendula Salve. *Skin Issue Salves*

Grapefruit, expressed, 22

Great Gardener Salve. *Salve*

GROWING YOUR OWN HERBS, 24

Guidelines for Using Herbs Safely, 39

Hanging Herbal Blends, 171

Headache Tea, 154

Hemorrhoid Liniment, 132

HERBS, 23

Herpes Helper Oil. *Infused Oil Blends*

Honey Dreams Bath, 81

Horseradish, 19

Hot Flash Massage oil, 57

Hot Flash- Massage Oil, 58

Hot Sex, 70

Household Cleaners. *Household Cleaners*

Hydrosol. *Extraction Methods of Essential Oils*

Immune Boost, 153

Impetigo, 142

In the Shower Inhalation. *Inhalation*

Indigestion, 57

Infant Massage Oil. *Medicinal Oils with Essential Oil*

Infused oil instructions. *Infused Oils*

Infused Oils, 41, 44

Infusion, 25

Infusion Herbs, 46

Inhalation, 35

Insect Remedies, 146

Insomnia Milk Bath, 81, *Bath Salts*

Intestinal Defense, 160

Iron Extract, 160

Itch-Away Spray, 147

Jaborandi, 19

Joint Care Blend, 161

Joyful Sensuality, 71

Kerchief Inhalation. *Inhalation*

Knee Oil, 49

Labor Massage Oil, 61

Labor Mists, 117

Lack of Energy Massage Oil, 69

Laundry Soap. *Household Cleaners*

Lavender Alcohol Based Bath Oil, 85

Lavender Infused Oil. *Infused Oil Blends*

Lavender Moisturizing Bubble Bath. *Bubble Bath*

Lavender Salt Scrub, 82

Lavender Shampoo, 144

Lavender vinegar lotion, 142

Lecithin Toner, 137

Left Over Scrub, 142

Lemon Fresh Sachets. *Fresh and Clean Sachet*

Lemon Toner, 139

Lemon, expressed, 22

Lime, expressed, 22

Linen Spray, 171

Linens, 171

Liniment Base, 129

LINIMENT OIL, 128

Liniments, 27

Lion Balm, 126

Lower Back Pain, 52

Lower Back Pain II, 52

Male Strength Tea, 153

Mama Milk, 150

Mama With a Cold Tea, 151

Mandarin, expressed, 22

Massage Oil (great for winter itch or nonspecific itching, 59

Massage Oil- Acute Inflammation, 51

Massage Oil for Common Colds, 54

Massage Oil for Dry Cough, 54

Massage Oil for Ear Infections, 55

Massage Oil for Feet, 55

Massage Oil for Feet 2, 55

Massage Oil for Gastric Headache, 56

Massage Oil for General Headache, 56

Massage Oil for Tendonitis, 50

Massage Oil for the Flu, 55

Massage Oil- Helpful with constipation pain, 57

Massage Oil Indigestion, 57

Massage Oil- Irritability, 69

Massage Oil- Lumbar Pain, 53

Massage Oil- Menstrual Cramps, 58

Melilotus, 20

Mellita, 30

Mellita Recipe, 30

Men's Health Glycerite Extract, 159

Menopause Massage oil, 57

Menopause- Night and Day Sweats, 58

Men's Tea, 152

Menstrual Cramp Oil, 58

Menstruation Sea Salt Bath. *Bath Salts*

Migraine Tea, 154

Milk and Honey Bath. *Bath Salts*

Milk Bath Salts. *BATH SALTS*

Milk Seed Tea, 151

Mint Bath. *Bath Salts*

Moisturizing Bubble Bath. *Bubble Bath*

Morning Sickness Oxymel, 157

Mosquito Repellent, 146

Moth Bag II. *Sachets*

Moth Bag Sachet. *Sachets*

Mother Anxiety, 151

Mother's Milk Tea, 152

Mud Baths, 90

Mugwort, 20

Murumuru Butter, 64

Muscle Relaxing Bath. *Bath Salts*

Muscle Soothing Tea, 90

Mustard, 20

My Favorite Football Liniment, 129

Natural Diaper Rash Balm, 126

Nerve Pain Oil, 53

Nerve Pain Salve, 122

Nervous System Tea. *Teas*

Nettle Herbal Hair Rinse, 146

No-Wax Linoleum Cleaner. *Household Cleaners*

Oatmeal and Almond Body Scrub, 83

Oatmeal Bath Salts. Bath Salts

Oatmeal Milk Bath. *BATH SALTS*

Oatmeal Therapeutic Bath Salts, 78

Oil, 43

Onion, 20

Outdoorsy Scent Potpourri. *Potpourri*

Oven Extraction. *Infused Oils*

Over The Bowl Inhalation. *Inhalation*

Overall Adrenal Support Extract, 161

Oxymel, 30

Pain Formula Extract, 161

Parsley Leaf, 22

Paste for Tennis Elbow, 135

Paste for Varicose Veins, 135

Pastes, 134

Pastes for Boils, 134

Pastes for Spots, 135

Patch testing skin, 9

Patch Testing the Environment, 9

Pennyroyal, 20

Peppermint Foot Scrub, 83

Petitgrain, 22

Pine Toner, 139

Pink Mud Bath. *See*

Pinks- Hanging Herbs, 171

Plantain Salve. *Skin Issue Salves*

Plaster. *Poultice*

Potpourri, 167

Poultice, 31

Poultice, Pulped. *Poultice*

Poultice, Steamed. *Poultice*

Pregnancy Oxymel, 157

Queen of Hungary Water, 140

Recipe Lingo!, 40

Refreshing Potpourri. *See*

Relaxation and Rest, 93

Relaxing Alcohol Based Bath Oil, 85

Relaxing Oil, 85

Revitalizing Oil, 84

Ring Worm, 142

Rinses, 133

Romantic Dreams Sachet. *Sachets*

Rose Alcohol Based Bath Oil, 85

Rose Water & Glycerin Astringent, 140

Rosemary Infused Oil. *Infused Oil Blends*

Rue, 20

Sachets, 168

Safety Tips for Essential Oils, 10

Sage Face Wash, 137

Sage Toner, 137

Salve, 34

Salves For What is Underneath, 122

Sassafras, 20

Sciatica. *Infused Oil Blends*

Sciatica Salve, 123

Sea Salt Body Polisher, 84

Sea Salts. *BATH SALTS*

Sensual Bath Oil, 84

Severe Eczema Blend. *Infused Oil Blends*

Sexy Cinnamon Tea, 155

Sexy Potpourri. Potpourri

Shampoo Base, 143

Shelf life. *Essential Oil Storage*

Shin Splints, 50

Shingles Oil, 56

Shingles Rinse, 134

Shingles Rinse II, 134

Shoe Freshener. *Household Cleaners*

Shoulder Tension Salve, 124

Sick wash. *Household Cleaners*

Simple Salve Instructions. *Salve*

Single Bath Oils, 87

Sinus Headache Bath Salts. *BATH SALTS*

Sinus Mist, 94

Skin Issue Massage Oils, 59

Skin Issue Salves, 120

Sleep Tea, 153

Sleepytime Bath Oil Blend, 86

Sleepytime Bed Linen, 172

Sleepytime Extract Blend, 161

Soapy Salt Scrub, 83

Solar infusion. *Infused Oils*

Soothing Bath Salts. *BATH SALTS*

Soothing Salve Recipe© Demetria Clark. *Salve*

Sore Muscle Alcohol Based Bath Oil, 86

Sore Muscle Bubble Bath. *Bubble Bath*

Sore Muscle Liniment, 129

Sore Muscle Oil. *Infused Oil Blends*

Sore Muscle Salve, 123

Sore Throat, 156

Southern Woods Sachet. *Sachets*

Spring Tonic, 155

St. John's Wort Salve. *Skin Issue Salves*

Stainless Steel Sink Cleaner. *Household Cleaners*

Stimulating Tea Bath, 89

Storing Herbs. *Herbs*

Stress Relief Tea, 90

Stress Relief Tea II, 90

Stretch Mark Balm, 125

Stretch Mark Massage Oil, 61

Sunshine Bubble Bath. *Bubble Bath*

Sunshine Towels, 172

Super Cleaning Spray. *Household Cleaners*

Super Sore Muscle Oil. *Infused Oil Blends*

Sweet Emotions Milk Bath. *BATH SALTS*

Sweet Sex, 70

Tagetes, 22

Tangerine, 22

Tansy, 20

Tea, 25

Tennis Elbow Oil, 50

Therapeutic Bath Salts, 77, *Bath Salts*

Throbbing Headache Tea, 154

Thuja, 21

Tick Repellent, 146

Tinctures, 29

Toilet Bowl Cleaner. *Household Cleaners*

Trouble Shooting Infused Oil Issues. *Infused Oils*

Tub scrub. *Household Cleaners*

Unsafe Oils, 18

Uplifting/Postpartum Blend, 94

Urinary Tract Ease, 154

Vanilla Bath Oil, 87

Varicose Vein Salve. *Salve*

Vein Oil, 54

Vitamin and Mineral Glycerite Extract, 159

Wildcrafting, 25

Willow Bark Pain Relief, 154

Window Cleaner. *Household Cleaners*

Window Wipes. *Household Cleaners*

Wintergreen, 21

Witch Hazel Liniment, 132

Women's Health Glycerite Extract, 159

Women's Tea, 152

Women's Tea II, 152

Wormseed, 21

Wormwood, 21

Yarrow Salve. *Skin Issue Salves*

YOU ROCK! Mamma Tea and Infusion, 150

Zit Zapper Toner, 138

Made in the USA
Lexington, KY
22 August 2014